Coping with Envy

DR WINDY DRYDEN was born in London in 1950. He has worked in psychotherapy and counselling for over 30 years, and is the author or editor of over 175 books, including *How to Accept Yourself* (Sheldon Press, 1999), *Self-discipline: How to get it and how to keep it* (Sheldon Press, 2009) and *Coping with Life's Challenges: Moving on from adversity* (Sheldon Press, 2010).

D1082593

Overcoming Common Problems Series

Selected titles

A full list of titles is available from Sheldon Press,
36 Causton Street, London SW1P 4ST and on our website at
www.sheldonpress.co.uk

Overcoming Common Problems Series

Overcoming Common Problems Series

Overcoming Common Problems

Coping with Envy

Feeling at a disadvantage with friends and family

DR WINDY DRYDEN

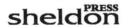

First published in Great Britain in 2010

Sheldon Press
36 Causton Street
London SW1P 4ST
www.sheldonpress.co.uk

Copyright © Dr Windy Dryden 2010

British Library Cataloguing-in-Publication Data

A catalogue record for this book is available from the British Library

ISBN 978–1–84709–102–4

1 3 5 7 9 10 8 6 4 2

Typeset by Fakenham Photosetting Ltd, Fakenham, Norfolk
Printed in Great Britain by Ashford Colour Press

Produced on paper from sustainable forests

Contents

1

Introduction

This book is based on the principles of Rational Emotive Behaviour Therapy (REBT), an approach to counselling that can be placed firmly in the cognitive–behavioural tradition of psychotherapy, meaning that it particularly focuses on the way that you think and behave when understanding your emotional response. REBT was founded in 1955 by Dr Albert Ellis, an American clinical psychologist who brought together his interests in philosophy and psychology, which are present in this approach over 55 years on. One of the hallmarks of REBT is that it holds that people can be taught and can learn the principles of good mental health.

In this book, then, I am working on the principle that I can teach you how to understand and discriminate between healthy and unhealthy envy, and how to address the factors that lead you to experience the latter so that you can end up by experiencing the former. Yes, that's right – it can be healthy to feel envious of a friend or family member! Such learning involves three stages: understanding, agreement and application.

First, you need to understand the factors that lead you to feel unhealthy envy and what you can do to overcome this troublesome emotion and become, where appropriate, healthily envious. If you don't understand the REBT model of unhealthy envy and its remediation that I outline in this book, then you will not be able to use it correctly to help yourself.

Second, you need to ask yourself whether or not you are in basic agreement with this model of unhealthy envy and its remediation. You may understand this model but not agree with it, in which case you will not use it to help yourself.

1

Third, you need to apply the model in your own life. This third step is perhaps the most important step of the three, for you may understand and agree with the REBT model of unhealthy envy and how it can be overcome, but unless you apply what you have learned you will not gain any real benefit from this book.

This point is so important, I want to reiterate it in a slightly different way. As writer and reader we have different responsibilities. My responsibility as author is to spell out the REBT model in as clear a way as I can and to outline how you can use it in practice, again as clearly as I am able. But you also have responsibilities as a reader, which can be analysed according to the understanding–agreement–application process that I have just put forward.

Thus, your first responsibility is to read this book carefully so that you can understand the REBT model of unhealthy envy and its remediation. Your second responsibility is to ask yourself whether or not you are in basic agreement with this model. This does not mean that you can't use this book unless you agree with everything that I have to say about unhealthy envy and how to cope with it. That would be far too black and white. Rather, it means that you need to agree with two basic premises: first, that unhealthy envy is based on an attitude of mind, and second, that you can deal constructively with your feelings of unhealthy envy by changing that attitude of mind and the behaviours that help to keep it alive. You may have a number of doubts, reservations and objections to some of the many detailed points that I will make, but if you are in broad agreement with the above two basic premises you can get a lot from this book.

However, you can only change the 'can' in that last statement to 'in all probability will' by discharging the third and the most important of your responsibilities: to apply what you have learned in this book. This application process warrants some brief discussion here although I will discuss it in greater detail later. I want to outline here that this application process involves you using the thinking and behavioural techniques that I will teach you in real-life settings, not just once or twice but repeatedly, until you begin to feel the benefit of them.

Unfortunately, emotional change (in this case from unhealthy envy to healthy envy) does not happen overnight, but is a long-drawn-out process that follows you rehearsing healthy beliefs and acting and thinking in ways that are consistent with these healthy beliefs. So if you are looking for a quick and effort-less fix, this book is decidedly not for you. However, if you are looking for a realistic approach to addressing your unhealthy envy based on deliberate practice of healthy ways of thinking and constructive ways of acting, then you may gain a lot from putting into practice the suggestions contained in these pages.

The same points listed above also apply when I discuss dealing with your own feelings, thinking and behaviour as the object of troublesome envy from a friend or family member. I will look at this issue in Chapter 5.

Let me now outline in general form the 'situational ABC' model that Albert Ellis, the founder of REBT, first introduced over 55 years ago. In reading this material, I want you to dis-charge your responsibilities for understanding the model and for ascertaining in your own mind whether or not you agree with the model.

The situational ABC model

Rational Emotive Behaviour Therapy (REBT) puts forward a straightforward 'situational ABC' model of psychological dis-turbance (which I will apply to unhealthy envy in Chapter 2). Let me outline this model in basic form before discussing each element in greater detail.

Situation

You do not react in a vacuum. Rather, you think, feel and act in specific situations. The 'situation' in the ABC refers to a descriptive account of the actual event to which you respond emotionally, behaviourally and cognitively.

'A' = activating event

Within this specific situation, when you have a significant emotional reaction it is usually to a key aspect of this situation. I refer to this as 'A', or the activating event, in this book.

'B' = belief

It is a major premise of REBT that while your emotions are usually about 'A', this 'A' does not cause the emotional reaction. Rather, your emotions are primarily determined by the beliefs that you hold about the 'A'.

'C' = consequences of the beliefs at 'B' about the activating event ('A')

When you hold a belief about the 'A', you will tend to experience an emotion, you will tend to act in a certain way and you will tend to think in certain ways. These three consequences of this 'A' × 'B' interaction are known as emotional, behavioural and thinking consequences, respectively.

Let me now discuss each of these elements in greater detail.

Situation

As I said earlier, emotional episodes do not take place in a vacuum. Rather, they occur in specific situations. Such situations are viewed in the situational ABC model as descriptions of actual events about which you form inferences (see below).

Situations can exist in time. Thus, they can describe past

actual events (e.g. 'My boss asked me to see her at the end of the day'), present actual events (e.g. 'My boss is asking me to see her at the end of the day') or future events (e.g. 'My boss will ask me to see her at the end of the day'). Note that I have not referred to such future events as future actual events since you don't know that such events will occur and this is why such future events may prove to be false. However, if you look at such future situations they are still descriptions of what may happen and do not add inferential meaning (see below).

Situations may refer to internal actual events (i.e. events that occur within yourself, such as thoughts, feelings, bodily sensations, aches and pains, etc.) or to external actual events (i.e. events that occur outside yourself, such as your boss asking to see you). Their defining characteristic is as before: they are descriptions of events and do not include inferential meaning.

'A'

As I said above, 'A' stands for activating event. This is the aspect of the situation about which you experience an emotional reaction. Let me make a number of points about 'A'.

An 'A' is usually an inference

An 'A' is usually an inference and needs to be differentiated from the situation or actual event about which it is made. An inference is basically an interpretation or hunch about the situation which goes beyond what can be described, whereas the situation is purely descriptive. Let me provide you with an example to make this distinction clear.

Imagine that you receive a message from your boss to the effect that she wants to see you at the end of the day. You think that this means she is going to criticize your work. The situation or actual event here is: 'My boss wants to see me at the end of the day', while your 'A' is: 'My boss is going to criticize my work.' As can be seen from this example, the situation is a description of the facts of the matter whereas the 'A' is the inferential aspect of the situation to which you have an emotional response.

Inferences that usually comprise the 'A' can be true or false

Inferences that usually comprise the 'A' can be true or false, and, as such, when you make an inference you need to evaluate it against the available evidence. Thus, in our example, it may be true that your boss is going to criticize your work when you go to see her at the end of the working day or it may be false. All you can do is to consider the available evidence and come up with the 'best bet' about what is going to happen at the meeting with the boss. This involves considering such factors as: (1) what has happened in the past when your boss has asked to see you; (2) the quality of the work that you recently submitted to your boss; and (3) how critical or otherwise your boss is in general.

An 'A' can be about a past, present or future event

When you have an 'A' about a past, present or future situation or actual event, you give that event inferential meaning. Thus:

Past situation = My boyfriend did not return my call.
'A' about past situation = This proves that he doesn't care for me.

Present situation = My phone is ringing and I can tell from the number display that it is my father.
'A' about present situation = My father is going to tell me off for overspending.

Future situation = The hospital will contact me with the results of my blood test.
'A' about future situation = The blood test will show that I am ill.

An 'A' can be about an event external to you or about an event internal to you

The defining characteristic of this 'A' is again its inferential nature. For example:

External situation = My letter with a cheque in it has gone missing.
'A' about external situation = Somebody has stolen my cheque.

Internal situation = I have an intrusive thought about hitting someone.
'A' about internal situation = I am losing control.

'B'

Beliefs are attitudes which can be rational (or healthy) or irrational (or unhealthy). You can hold beliefs about descriptive situations, but more often you will hold beliefs about the 'A's that you make about these more objective situations. I will begin by discussing rational beliefs.

Rational beliefs

REBT argues that there are four basic rational beliefs. I will outline them very shortly and return to them when I come to discuss healthy envy in Chapter 3. Before I do so, let me just say that rational beliefs have five major characteristics. They are:

1 flexible or non-extreme;
2 conducive to your mental health;
3 helpful to you as you strive towards your goals;
4 true;
5 logical.

Now let me discuss the four rational beliefs put forward by REBT theory.

Non-dogmatic preference

Human beings have desires, and for desires to be the cornerstone of healthy functioning they need to take the form of a non-dogmatic preference. This has two components. The first component is called the 'asserted preference' component. Here, you make clear to yourself what you want (either what you want to happen or exist, or what you want not to happen or exist). The second component is called the 'negated demand' component. Here, you acknowledge that what you want to occur or exist does not have to occur or exist.

In short, we have:

Non-dogmatic preference = asserted preference component + negated demand component.

Non-awfulizing belief

When your non-dogmatic preference is not met, it is healthy for you to conclude that it is bad that you have not got what you want. It is not healthy to be indifferent about not getting what you desire. As with a non-dogmatic preference, a non-awfulizing belief has two components. The first component may be called the 'asserted badness' component. Here, you acknowledge that it is bad that you have not got what you want or that you have got what you don't want. The second component is called the 'anti-awfulizing' component. Here, you acknowledge that while it is bad when you don't get your desires met it is not awful, terrible or the end of the world.

In short, we have:

Non-awfulizing belief = asserted badness component + anti-awfulizing component.

High frustration tolerance (HFT) belief

When your non-dogmatic preference is not met, it is healthy for you to conclude that it is difficult for you to tolerate not getting what you want but that you can tolerate it. An HFT belief also has three components. The first component may be called the 'asserted struggle' component because you recognize that it is a struggle to put up with not getting what you want. The second component is called the 'negated unbearability' component. Here, you acknowledge that while it is a struggle to tolerate not getting your desires met, it is not intolerable. The third component is called the 'worth tolerating' component and points to the fact that not only can you tolerate not getting what you want, but it is worth doing so.

In short, we have:

High frustration tolerance belief = asserted struggle component + negated unbearability component + worth tolerating component.

Acceptance belief

When your non-dogmatic preference is not met, it is healthy for you to accept this state of affairs. There are three types of acceptance belief: a 'self-acceptance' belief where you accept yourself for not meeting your desires or for not having them met; an 'other-acceptance' belief where you accept another person or other people for not meeting your desires; and an 'acceptance of life conditions' belief where you accept life conditions when they don't meet your desires.

There are three components to an acceptance belief which I will illustrate with reference to a self-acceptance belief. The first component is called the 'negatively evaluated aspect' component. Here, you recognize when you have not met your desires or when your desires have not been met by others or by life conditions, and you evaluate this particular aspect negatively. The second component is called the 'negated global negative evaluation' component. Here, you acknowledge that while you may have acted badly, for example, or experienced a bad event, the whole of you is not bad. It proves that you are a complex fallible human being, which is the third component, called the 'asserted complex fallibility' component.

In short, we have:

Acceptance belief = negatively evaluated aspect component + negated global negative evaluation component + asserted complex fallibility component.

Irrational beliefs

REBT argues that there are four basic irrational beliefs. I will outline them very shortly and return to them when I come to discuss unhealthy envy in Chapter 2. Before I do so, let me just say that irrational beliefs have five major characteristics. They are:

1 rigid or extreme;
2 conducive to psychological disturbance;
3 unhelpful to you as you strive towards your goals;
4 false;
5 illogical.

Now let me discuss the four irrational beliefs put forward by REBT theory.

Demand

REBT theory holds that when you take your desires and turn them into rigid demands, absolute necessities, musts, absolute shoulds and the like, you make yourself emotionally disturbed when you don't get what you believe you must. Even when you do get what you believe you must, you are still vulnerable to emotional disturbance if you hold a rigid demand at the point where you become aware that you might lose what you have and believe you need.

A rigid demand has two components. The first is known as the 'asserted preference' component and is the same as the asserted preference component of a non-dogmatic preference. Again, here you make clear to yourself what you want (either what you want to happen or exist or what you want not to happen or exist). The second component is called the 'asserted demand' component. Here, you take what you want and you turn it into a 'rigid demand' (e.g. 'I want to do well in my examination and therefore I have to do so').

In short, we have:

Rigid demand = asserted preference component + asserted demand component.

Awfulizing belief

When your rigid demand is not met, then you will tend to reach the extreme conclusion that it is awful, horrible, terrible or the end of the world that you haven't got what you insist you must have. As with an non-awfulizing belief, an awfulizing belief has two components. The first component is the same as that in the non-awfulizing belief – the 'asserted badness' component. Here, you acknowledge that it is bad that you have not got what you want or that you have got what you don't want. The second component is called the 'asserted awfulizing' component. Here, you transform your non-extreme evaluation of badness into an extreme evaluation of horror (e.g. 'Because it would be bad if I were to fail my exam, it would be horrible were I to do so').

In short, we have:

Awfulizing belief = asserted badness component + asserted awfulizing component.

Low frustration tolerance (LFT) belief

When your rigid demand is not met, you will tend to make the extreme conclusion that you can't bear not getting what you demand. Unlike an HFT belief, which has three components, an LFT belief tends to have only two components. The first component is again known as the 'asserted struggle' component, because you recognize that it is a struggle to put up with not getting what you believe you must get. The second component is called the 'asserted unbearability' component. Here, you acknowledge that it is not just a struggle to put up with not getting your demand met, it is intolerable. Since you think that you cannot put up with not getting your demand met, the issue of whether or not it is worth tolerating does not become an issue. You can't tolerate it and that's that.

In short, we have:

Low frustration tolerance belief = asserted struggle component + asserted unbearability component.

Depreciation belief

When your rigid demands are not met, you will tend to depreciate yourself, depreciate others or depreciate life conditions. Thus, there are three types of depreciation belief: a self-depreciation belief where you depreciate yourself for not meeting your demands or for not having them met; an other-depreciation belief where you depreciate another person or other people for not meeting your demands; and a depreciation of life conditions belief where you depreciate life conditions when they don't meet your demands.

There are two components to a depreciation belief which I will illustrate with reference to a self-depreciation belief. The first component is called the 'negatively evaluated aspect' component. Here, you recognize that you have not met your demands or that your demands have not been met by others or by life conditions, and you evaluate this particular aspect negatively. The second component is called the 'asserted global negative evaluation' component. Here, you give yourself a global negative rating for not meeting your demands, for example. Thus, you may acknowledge that you have acted badly and then evaluate yourself as a bad person for acting badly.

In short, we have:

Depreciation belief = negatively evaluated aspect component + asserted global negative evaluation component.

'C'

'C' stands for the consequences that you experience when you hold a belief at 'B' about 'A'. There are three major consequences, which I will consider separately but which in reality occur together.

Emotional 'C's

When your 'A' is negative and you hold a set of rational beliefs at 'B' about this 'A', your emotional 'C' will be negative, but healthy. Yes, that's right – negative emotions can be healthy. Thus, when you face a threat it is healthy to feel concerned, and when you have experienced a loss it is healthy to feel sad. Other healthy negative emotions (so called because they feel unpleasant but help you to deal constructively with negative life events) are: remorse, disappointment, sorrow, healthy anger, healthy jealousy and healthy envy.

When your 'A' is negative but this time you hold a set of irrational beliefs at 'B' about this 'A', your emotional 'C' will be negative and unhealthy. Thus, when you face a threat it is unhealthy to feel anxious, and when you have experienced a loss it is unhealthy to feel depressed. Other unhealthy negative emotions (so called because they feel unpleasant and they interfere with you dealing constructively with negative life events) are: guilt, shame, hurt, unhealthy anger, unhealthy jealousy and unhealthy envy (the subject of this book).

Behavioural 'C's

When your 'A' is negative and you hold a set of rational beliefs at 'B' about this 'A', your behavioural 'C' is likely to be constructive. Such behaviour is constructive in three ways. First, it will help you to change the negative event that you are facing if it can be changed. Second, it will help you to make a healthy adjustment if the event cannot be changed, and third, it will help you to go forward and make progress at achieving your goals.

When your 'A' is negative but this time you hold a set of irrational beliefs at 'B' about this 'A', your behavioural 'C' will be unconstructive. Such behaviour is unconstructive, again in three ways. First, it won't help you to change the negative event that you are facing if it can be changed. Indeed, such unconstructive behaviour will often make a bad situation worse. Second, it will prevent you from making a healthy adjustment if the event cannot be changed, and third, it will take you away from pursuing your goals.

Thinking 'C's

When your 'A' is negative and you hold a set of rational beliefs at 'B' about this 'A', your subsequent thinking (or thinking 'C's) is likely to be constructive. Such thinking is constructive in two ways. First, it is realistic and allows you to deal with probable outcomes. Second, it is balanced and recognizes, for example, that you will get a range of positive, neutral and negative responses to your behaviour. As a result these thinking 'C's enable you to respond constructively to realistically perceived situations.

When your 'A' is negative but this time you hold a set of irrational beliefs at 'B' about this 'A', your subsequent thinking (or thinking 'C's) is likely to be unconstructive. Such thinking is unconstructive in two ways. First, it is unrealistic in that you will tend to over-predict the existence of low-probability, highly aversive outcomes. Second, it is skewed in that you think, for example, that most people will respond to you negatively, a few may respond to you neutrally but nobody will respond to you positively. As a result these thinking 'C's interfere with your ability to respond constructively to realistically perceived situations.

Summary

Let me summarize what I have discussed in this section in dia-grammatic form:

Situational ABC of psychological health

Situation = Objectively described event.

'A' = Aspect of the situation to which your respond emotionally, behaviourally and cognitively.

'B' = Rational belief
- Non-dogmatic preference
- Non-awfulizing belief
- High frustration tolerance belief
- Acceptance belief.

'C' = Consequences
- Emotional (healthy negative)
- Behavioural (constructive)
- Thinking (realistic and balanced).

Situational ABC of psychological disturbance

Situation = Objectively described event.

'A' = Aspect of the situation to which you respond emotionally, behaviourally and cognitively.

'B' = Rational belief
- Rigid demand
- Awfulizing belief
- Low frustration tolerance belief
- Depreciation belief.

'C' = Consequences
- Emotional (unhealthy negative)
- Behavioural (unconstructive)
- Thinking (unrealistic and skewed).

Other issues

Before closing this chapter I wish to discuss three other issues: (1) the two domains of envy; (2) the two different types of envy; and (3) the envy grid. I will introduce these ideas here and will expand on them in the rest of the book.

The two domains of envy

There are two domains of envy: the ego domain of envy and the non-ego domain of envy. In the ego domain of envy, your envy is related to how you view yourself, while in the non-ego domain of envy your envy is not related to how you view yourself

The two different types of envy

Earlier, I distinguished between healthy negative emotions (which stem from rational beliefs) and unhealthy negative emotions (which stem from irrational beliefs). Thus, there are two different types of envy: healthy envy and unhealthy envy. In this book. I will be helping you to address and cope with unhealthy envy and to experience healthy envy when appropriate.

The envy grid

If we put the above two concepts together, we have the envy grid with the following four elements:

- Healthy ego envy
- Healthy non-ego envy
- Unhealthy ego envy
- Unhealthy non-ego envy.

I will explain and expand on these in the appropriate chapters of this book. In the next chapter, I will discuss the ABCs of unhealthy envy.

2

The ABCs of unhealthy envy

Introduction

In this chapter, I will consider what people tend to be unhealthily envious about and discuss the irrational beliefs that underpin unhealthy envy. In doing so, I will focus on envy among family and friends. I will also consider what people tend to do and think when they experience unhealthy envy, and will show how these forms of behaviour and thinking serve to maintain unhealthy envy. I will use the ABC framework discussed in Chapter 1 to structure the material.

As you read this chapter, I want you to remember a point that I outlined in the first chapter: that there are two main types of envy, unhealthy envy and healthy envy. In this chapter I will focus on unhealthy envy and will discuss healthy envy in the following chapter.

What you feel unhealthily envious about

In this section I will consider what people are generally unhealthily envious about with respect to their family and friends.

Theme and components

There is one key theme that appears in people's descriptions of what they envy in family members and friends. This theme is present no matter what you envy and no matter whether your envy is healthy or unhealthy. The theme is as follows:

> You feel envious (healthily or unhealthily) about someone else having that which you prize but do not possess.

Let me break this down into its component parts before I discuss the content of your envy.

- You.
- Someone else. (This can be one person or a group of people. For our purposes in this book, it can be a family member or a friend.)
- Something that you prize. (As we will see, what you prize can be quite varied.)
- The other possesses what you prize and do not have: this is the central component of all envy.

As I noted above, what you envy can be very varied and depends very much on your idiosyncratic desires. Without attempting to be comprehensive, let me list some of the major things you may envy – what a family member or friend has that you do not possess.

- A material possession or possessions
- Lifestyle (including wealth)
- A personality characteristic
- A physical characteristic
- A relationship or relationships
- Social attention and/or recognition
- Public awards or honours
- Status and/or power.

Object-focused unhealthy envy

Envy can be largely object-focused or person-focused. When your envy is object-focused your focus is on the 'object' (a generic term for all the items listed above) that another has and that you don't have, rather than on the person who has it. Thus, this type of envy is called object-focused envy because what you envy is more relevant than who you envy. In its unhealthy form, this type of envy is called object-focused unhealthy envy.

I will now turn my attention to person-focused envy, or who you tend to unhealthily envy.

Who you tend to unhealthily envy

When unhealthy envy is largely person-focused, your focus is on the person rather than on the 'object' (or what the person has). Generally speaking, in person-focused unhealthy envy, the family member or friend whom you envy is often (but not always) someone (1) to whom you consider yourself to be inferior and/or (2) whom you consider to be a rival. This explains why you may feel unhealthily envious when your sister has something that you prize but don't have, but not envious at all when your cousin has that very same 'object'. When the 'who' is more important than the 'what', this type of envy is called person-focused envy. In its unhealthy form it is known as person-focused unhealthy envy.

Why you feel unhealthily envious

So far I have discussed the major theme in envy (that someone else has something that you desire, but lack) and I have considered both what and who you envy. None of these factors, however, get to the core of the 'why' question, i.e. why you have feelings of unhealthy envy. To answer this question we need to return to the situational ABC framework and to use an example. Let's suppose that you and a friend go for the same job; he gets the job and you feel unhealthily envious. Using the situational ABC framework, we have the following:

Situation = My friend and I both went for a job, which he got.
'A' = He has the job that I wanted but didn't get.
'B' = ?
'C' = Unhealthy envy.

According to REBT theory, as I discussed in the first chapter, while your emotions are influenced by situations and, in particular, the inferences that you make about these situations (at 'A'), neither these situations nor the inferences at 'A' determine your emotions. Rather, it is the beliefs that you hold about these situations and, in particular, about the inferences that you form about the situations that have a much greater determining effect on the way that you feel (and the way that you act and subsequently think, for that matter). If you hold a set of rational beliefs (at 'B') about negative situations and inferences (at 'A') then your feelings (at 'C') will be healthy and negative. However, if your beliefs are irrational in the same set of circumstances then your feelings will be unhealthy and negative.

Since the example that I have provided shows that you feel unhealthily envious, we can assume that your beliefs at B are irrational. I will now discuss these irrational beliefs in the context of four types of unhealthy envy. These are:

- Unhealthy ego envy: object-focused
- Unhealthy non-ego envy: object-focused
- Unhealthy ego envy: person-focused
- Unhealthy non-ego envy: person-focused.

While in practice your unhealthy envy may have elements of one or more of these different types, I will here consider them in their pure form.

Unhealthy ego envy: object-focused

In this type of unhealthy envy, your focus is on the job that your friend got and that you wanted but didn't get. Since your unhealthy envy is ego in nature, your irrational beliefs reflect this, as in the following:

Situation = My friend and I both went for a job, which he got.
'A' = Not having *a job* like the one my friend got.

'B' = I must have *a job* like the one he has. (Demand)
I am less worthy because I don't have *a job* like the one he has.
(Self-depreciation belief)
'C' = Unhealthy envy.

Note the following in the above ABC analysis:

1 In 'A', the emphasis is on the job and not the person who has the job. It is likely, therefore, that you may have felt unhealthily envious if someone else had got the job and you hadn't.
2 I have concentrated on your demand and self-depreciation belief, since these are the most salient in unhealthy ego envy.

Unhealthy non-ego envy: object-focused

In this type of unhealthy envy, your focus is again on the job that your friend got and that you wanted but didn't get. Since your unhealthy envy is non-ego in nature, your irrational beliefs reflect this, as in the following:

Situation = My friend and I both went for a job, which he got.
'A' = Not having *a job* like the one my friend got.
'B' = I must have *a job* like the one he has. (Demand)
It's terrible that I don't have *a job* like the one my friend got.
(Awfulizing belief)
I can't bear being deprived of what I want, i.e. *a job* like the one he got. (Low frustration tolerance belief)
'C' = Unhealthy envy.

Note the following in the above ABC analysis:

1 In 'A', the emphasis is again on the job and not the person who has the job. It is again likely that you might have felt unhealthily envious if someone else had got the job and you hadn't.
2 I have concentrated on your demand, awfulizing and LFT beliefs since these are the most salient in unhealthy non-ego envy. However, in future when I discuss unhealthy non-ego envy I will feature either an awfulizing belief or an

LFT belief, since the demand and one of these beliefs are usually sufficient to account for this type of unhealthy envy.

Unhealthy ego envy: person-focused

In this type of unhealthy envy, your focus is on the person who has the job rather than on the job itself. Since your unhealthy envy is ego in nature, your irrational beliefs reflect this, as in the following:

Situation = My friend and I both went for a job, which he got.
'A' = *My friend* having something (a job) that I don't have, but want.
'B' = *He* must not have what I don't have. (Demand)
The fact that *he* has what I don't have means that I am less worthy than he is. (Self-depreciation belief)
'C' = Unhealthy envy.

Note the following in the above ABC analysis:

1 In 'A', the emphasis is on the person and not on the job. It is likely, therefore, that you may feel unhealthily envious towards this person for other things he may have that you lack, whereas you may not feel unhealthily envious towards another person who got the job rather than you.
2 I have once again concentrated on your demand and self-depreciation belief since these are the most salient in unhealthy ego envy.

Unhealthy non-ego envy: person-focused

In this type of unhealthy envy, your focus is once again on the person and not on the job. Since your unhealthy envy is non-ego in nature, your irrational beliefs reflect this, as in the following:

Situation = My friend and I both went for a job, which he got.
'A' = It is unfair that *he* got the job that I wanted and didn't get.
'B' = This unfairness where *my friend* got what I wanted absolutely should not exist. (Demand)

It is terrible that this unfairness where *he* got what I wanted
has occurred. (Awfulizing belief)
'C' = Unhealthy envy.

Note the following in the above ABC analysis:

1 In 'A', the emphasis is on the unfairness that this person got
the job rather than on the unfairness that you didn't get the
job. It is likely that you would feel unhealthily envious if this
named person experiences other unfair (as deemed by you)
advantages.
2 I have concentrated on your demand and awfulizing belief
here. I could also have focused on your demand and LFT
belief.

Before I leave the irrational beliefs that are at the core of your
feelings of unhealthy envy, I want to stress that these irrational
beliefs may take one of two major forms. While both of these
irrational beliefs are about someone else having what you covet
but don't have, they differ in one major respect. One set of
unhealthy envy-based irrational beliefs focuses on you and you
getting what you covet (e.g. 'I must have what he has'). Here,
you are satisfied, albeit temporarily, if you get what you demand.
The other set of unhealthy envy-related irrational beliefs focuses
on the other person and what he or she has in relation to what
you do not have (e.g. 'She must not have what I do not have').
Here you would be satisfied, again temporarily, were that person
to lose what you covet.

How you think when you feel unhealthily envious

When you hold a set of unhealthy envy-related irrational
beliefs, these beliefs will influence how you subsequently think.
These thoughts tend to be elaborations on the unhealthy envy
theme, and/or are relevant inferences and/or are action-related.

Thinking about how to get what you envy regardless of its usefulness, attainability and the cost of pursuing it

When you are unhealthily envious because you demand that you must get what your friend or family member has that you lack, then you will tend to think about whatever it is that you covet but don't have. Your thoughts will not only concern the 'object' but will also be about how to get it. When your thoughts are in this direction, you tend not to think of the usefulness of the 'object', whether it is attainable or the price that you may have to pay (financially and psychologically) in your pursuit of it. This type of thinking is particularly a feature of object-focused unhealthy envy (see pp. 20–22).

Thinking about depriving the other person of what you envy

When your unhealthy envy-related irrational belief is focused on what your friend or family member has in relation to what you do not have, then this belief will encourage you to think about ways in which you can deprive the person of his or her coveted 'object'. This type of thinking is particularly a feature of person-focused unhealthy envy (see pp. 22–3).

Thinking that not having what you want is unfair whether it is unfair or not

As I mentioned earlier in this book, unhealthy envy concerns an imbalanced situation where a friend or family member has something that you do not have but covet. You covet this 'object' either because you want it or because you are envious of the other person, in which case you covet the 'object' not because you necessarily want it *per se* but because the envied other person has it.

Now, when you hold an unhealthy envy-related irrational belief about this situation, which is to you imbalanced, this irrational belief will encourage you to see this situation as dreadfully unfair. This will be the case whether it is objectively unfair or not. Indeed, you may have every conceivable advantage and still think it is dreadfully unfair to not have an 'object' that you covet when you hold an unhealthy envy-related irrational belief.

Once you have created this unfairness in your mind, you can focus on it as a new 'A' and then disturb yourself about it by using a further set of irrational beliefs. The resultant feelings of self-pity and/or resentment often accompany unhealthy envy, as I will discuss in Chapter 5.

Thoughts of unfairness can help you to justify thinking about ways of depriving the other person of what you covet, as discussed in the above section. Thus, if you think that it is very unfair that a friend was given promotion over you (thinking consequence of a prior unhealthy envy-related irrational belief), then when you plot and scheme in your mind about how to get her sacked from her new position, you can justify your scheming to yourself because of the great unfairness that has befallen you.

Thinking about spoiling or destroying what you covet so that the other person does not have it

I described above how unhealthy envy-related irrational beliefs lead you to have thoughts of how to deprive your family member or friend of what you covet (either because you truly covet the 'object' or because you are unhealthily envious of the person who happens to have what you don't have). These irrational beliefs can also lead you to have thoughts of spoiling or even destroying a coveted 'object' that another person has (again, either because you truly covet the 'object' or because you are envious of the other person who has the 'object'). Thus, when under the influence of an unhealthy envy-related irrational belief, you might think of spoiling your sister's new car by scratching it with a sharp knife when nobody is around or (more seriously) you may think of ways of destroying it altogether.

Thinking denigrating thoughts about what you covet

Many of the thinking consequences of unhealthy envy-based irrational beliefs that I have already discussed in this chapter are cognitive attempts to eradicate a basic perceived inequality. This is particularly the case when you think denigrating thoughts about what you covet, whether you really covet it or whether you do so because the family member or friend whom you envy has it. This is known as the 'sour grapes' mentality. Thus, if you hold unhealthy envy-based irrational beliefs about the fact that a family member or friend has 'grapes' that you covet but don't have, then you may remove the inequality of not having what you believe you must have and therefore feel better (albeit temporarily) by telling yourself that the 'grapes' are sour. While this thinking consequence can be found in both person-focused and object-focused unhealthy envy, it is particularly associated with the latter, since you are denigrating the 'object' rather than the family member or friend who has the 'object'.

Thinking denigrating thoughts about the person you envy

When the focus of your unhealthy envy is a family member or friend rather than an 'object' that someone has, then a thinking consequence of the irrational beliefs that underpin such unhealthy envy involves you thinking denigrating thoughts about the family member or friend whom you envy. This is a common thinking method of making things equal in your mind.

Convincing yourself that you are happy with what you have

Another way of making things equal in your mind, once you hold a set of unhealthy envy-based irrational beliefs, is to try to convince yourself that you are happy with what you have in life. If you can convince yourself that you are happy with your lot in life, then you have made things equal in your mind. However, this thinking strategy involves a fair measure of self-deception if it is to be successful, and you may not be able to do this, particularly if you have previously admitted to yourself that you feel unhealthily envious.

Thinking that you won't try to get the coveted 'object' even though you really want it

When you hold an unhealthy envy-related irrational belief, you may think that there is no point in trying to get the 'object' that you covet but don't have because you think that there is no chance of getting it. This holds even if you would gain enduring use and/or enjoyment of the 'object' under consideration. Irrational beliefs tend to lead to 'all or nothing' thinking, and therefore if you are not sure that you will get the coveted 'object' then you will think that you will never get it. Since you think you will never get it, then it makes sense, in your mind, not even to try for it.

Thinking consequences of holding unhealthy envy-based irrational beliefs can be obsessive

So far, I have discussed the thinking consequences of holding unhealthy envy-based irrational beliefs in their most commonly occurring non-obsessive form. However, if you have a tendency to obsessive thinking, you may bring this tendency to these thinking consequences and end up making yourself even more disturbed. The hallmark of obsessive thinking is its repetitive nature and a sense that these thoughts have a life of their own. Thus, having made yourself feel unhealthily envious by holding one or more unhealthy envy-related irrational beliefs, you may obsessively think:

- of ways to get what you covet;
- of ways to deprive your friend or family member of what he or she has that you covet;
- of ways to spoil or destroy what the friend or family member has;
- of the unfairness of the situation where your friend or family member has what you covet but do not have;
- denigrating thoughts of what you covet;
- denigrating thoughts of the friend or family member whom you unhealthily envy.

If your obsessive unhealthy envy-related thoughts interfere with your working and/or personal life, I suggest that you contact your GP to discuss with him or her whether you should seek professional help.

How you act (or tend to act) when you feel unhealthily envious

So far I have considered:

- what you make yourself unhealthily envious about (usually a friend or family member having something that you want but don't have, and where the focus is either on the 'object' itself or the friend or family member who has the 'object');
- how you make yourself unhealthily envious (by holding one or more irrational beliefs about the above situation);
- the thinking consequences of holding these unhealthy envy-based irrational beliefs.

In this section, I will consider the behavioural consequences of holding unhealthy envy-related irrational beliefs. Before I do so, I want to make two points:

1 The behavioural consequences of unhealthy envy-related irrational beliefs can be either urges to act (sometimes known

as action tendencies) or actual actions. Suffice it to say, when you experience an unhealthy envy-related urge to act you have a choice. You can either resist acting on it or you can, of course, act on it.

2 Unhealthy envy-related behavioural consequences are frequently the behavioural expressions of the thinking consequences of holding unhealthy envy-related irrational beliefs. In this way, thinking and behaviour often go together. However, they do not have to go together and, in the same way as you don't have to act on your unhealthy envy-related action tendency, you don't have to act on your unhealthy envy-related thinking.

When you hold a set of unhealthy envy-related irrational beliefs, you then act or tend to act in one or more of the following ways:

Seeking out what you envy whether you really want it or not

When your unhealthy irrational beliefs are object-focused, then you will tend to seek out what you covet and often spend an inordinate amount of time trying to get it, sometimes going well out of your way to get it. This tends to be the case whether or not you truly want the 'object' in question. If you do truly want it, your irrational belief then turns that desire into an absolute necessity, and means that while you are motivated to get what you covet you pursue getting it in a desperate manner and are very anxious in case you don't succeed in getting it. If you don't truly want it – which is often the case in unhealthy envy based on the idea that you must not be deprived of something that a friend or family member has, and in person-focused unhealthy envy where you think you want something that a friend or family member whom you unhealthily envy has (when in reality you don't) – then your frantic efforts to get the 'object' in question are particularly self-defeating, since you are pursuing something that intrinsically you don't really want.

Casting aside what you envy once you have got it

When you hold a set of unhealthy envy-based irrational beliefs, what you are really demanding is either (1) equality, where you get what you covet, or (2) an end to inequality, where you deprive your friend or family member of what you covet. When you hold an unhealthy envy-based irrational belief and you gain equality by getting what you covet, then, because your real agenda is equality rather than obtaining the 'object' itself, you will quickly cast aside the 'object' in question. This is particularly the case in person-focused unhealthy envy. Even when you get an 'object' that you truly want, when you hold an unhealthy envy-based irrational belief you will also cast this 'object' aside as soon as you become aware of some other inequality where yet another friend or family member has something that you value but don't have.

This behavioural consequence of unhealthy envy-based irrational beliefs helps to explain why, if you are particularly prone to unhealthy envy, you are rarely, if ever, satisfied with what you have, because you are preoccupied with what you don't have and, as soon as soon as you get what you don't have, you shift your attention to something else that your friends or family members have that you don't have.

Other actions that stem from unhealthy envy-related irrational beliefs are behavioural expressions of the thinking consequences of these beliefs discussed above. These are:

- actively attempting to take away what you covet from a friend or family member;
- actively striving to spoil or destroy your friend's or family member's coveted 'object';
- verbally disparaging to others the friend or family member whom you unhealthily envy, and encouraging these others to disparage this person;

- verbally disparaging to others the 'object' that you unhealthily envy and encouraging them to disparage the 'object';
- telling others that you don't really want what you do, in truth, covet;
- not trying to get the coveted 'object' even though you really want it, because you think that there is no chance of getting it.

When you are prone (and not prone) to unhealthy envy

If you experience unhealthy envy, it is important for you to determine how prone you are to this destructive emotion. When you experience unhealthy envy infrequently in a small number of specific situations, then you can be said not to be particularly prone to unhealthy envy. On the other hand, if you experience unhealthy envy frequently in a great number of situations then you can be said to be prone to unhealthy envy.

When you are particularly prone to unhealthy envy, the following is likely to be the case:

- You frequently focus on 'objects' that you don't have but covet, and on the iniquitous nature of you not possessing what your friends and/or family members possess.
- You frequently harbour feelings of unhealthy envy towards friends and/or family members.
- Your unhealthy envy-based irrational beliefs occupy a core place in your belief system.
- You operate on one or more of the following core irrational beliefs:
  - Your worth is dependent on having what friends and family members have in life.
  - Friends and family members whom you envy are more worthwhile than you.
  - The inequality of friends and family members having what

you don't have is intolerable and such inequality must not be allowed to exist.

– You must have what you want and it is awful to be deprived.

- You frequently focus on the unfairness (as you see it) of not having what friends and/or family members have and rarely focus on the unfairness of having what friends and/or family members do not have.

- You frequently think of ways of getting even with friends and/or family members, either by getting what they have or by spoiling or depriving them of what they have. You either act on these thoughts or 'feel' like acting on them.

- You frequently attempt to equalize things in your mind by disparaging 'objects' you covet that friends and/or family members have and/or by disparaging these envied people. You may do this just in your mind and/or you may voice your disparaging views to others and attempt to elicit their agreement with your views. When you are successful in this, you may engage in mutual disparaging with those individuals and seek them out for regular 'bitching' sessions.

- In my book *How to Make Yourself Miserable* (Sheldon Press, 2001), I show that when you are prone to unhealthy envy you operate on a view of the world that is founded on the irrational beliefs that underpin this emotion. The following are the major components of the unhealthy envy-based world view and the inferences that you tend to make when you operate on this world view.

  – 'The grass is always greener in the lives of my friends and/or family members' ('Whatever I have is less attractive than what my friends and/or family members have').

  – 'I can only be satisfied if I get what I want' ('If I get what I covet it will satisfy me').

  – 'It's unfair if friends and/or family have what I don't have, but it is fair if I have what they don't have' ('If I don't have something that I covet, but lack, this inequality is unfair').

- 'People's worth is defined by what they have in life' ('People will like me more if I have a lot in my life than if I have a little').
- 'The more I have, the happier I'll be' ('In any situation it is better to have what I don't have than to be content with what I do have').

However, when you are *not* particularly prone to unhealthy envy, the following is likely to be the case:

- You will also focus on 'objects' that you don't have but covet, and on the iniquitous nature of you not possessing what friends and/or family members possess, but you will do so infrequently and in circumscribed situations.
- You will infrequently feel unhealthy envy towards your friends and/or family members.
- Your unhealthy envy-based irrational beliefs are situational and do not occupy a core place in your belief system.
- You may believe in the following non-core, situationally held irrational beliefs:
  - Your worth is dependent on having what a few specific friends and/or family members have in life.
  - A few specific friends or family members are more worth-while than you.
  - The inequality of a small number of specific friends and/or family members having what you don't have is intolerable and such inequality must not be allowed to exist.
  - You must have a small number of specific 'objects' that you want and it is awful to be deprived.
- However, you do *not* generally believe that:
  - your worth is dependent on having what a broad range of friends and family members have in life;

  – a broad range of friends and family members are more worthwhile than you;
  – the inequality of friends and family members having what you don't have is intolerable and such inequality must not be allowed to exist;
  – you must have what you want and it is awful to be deprived.

- You only focus on the unfairness (as you see it) of not having what friends and/or family members have in a small number of specific situations.

- You only think of ways of getting even with friends and/or family members, either by getting what they have or by spoiling or depriving them of what they have, in a small number of specific situations. You only act on these thoughts or 'feel' like acting on them in these specific contexts.

- You only attempt to equalize things in your mind by disparaging 'objects' you covet that friends and/or family friends have or by disparaging such envied people in a small number of specific situations, and only act on these thoughts infrequently and in a limited number of specific situations.

- You tend not to have a world view based on unhealthy envy since you only experience this destructive emotion in specific situations.

In this book, I will first help you to deal with specific episodes of unhealthy envy whether or not you are particularly prone to it. Then, if you are particularly prone to unhealthy envy, I will help you to become less prone to this destructive emotion.

Why you may be reluctant to deal with your feelings of unhealthy envy

There are two important steps to take before you can deal constructively with an emotional problem. The first step is to admit to yourself that you have the problem, and the second step is to take responsibility for factors within your control that have led to the problem. Now, you may be reluctant to deal with your feelings of unhealthy envy because you won't take one or both of these steps. Let's consider some of the reasons why you may not do so.

Denying to yourself that you feel unhealthily envious

Why might you not admit to yourself that you are unhealthily envious when, in truth, you do experience these feelings? One reason is that you feel ashamed of these feelings. As I showed in my book *Overcoming Shame* (Sheldon Press, 1997), one of the effects of feeling ashamed about your feelings is to deny to yourself and to your friends and/or family members that you have such feelings. You do this because you hold a version of the following irrational belief: 'I must not feel this way and if I do it proves that I am a weak, defective or disgraceful person.' I hope you can see that if you hold such a belief about feeling unhealthily envious, then it will be difficult for you to own up to having such feelings. Also, academic research has shown that unhealthy envy is generally regarded in many cultures as one of the most shameful of emotions to experience. So, as there is a cultural taboo about experiencing unhealthy envy, this would be another reason you may find it difficult to admit to yourself that you feel unhealthily envious.

If you do feel ashamed about feeling unhealthy envy, you will need to overcome your shame before fully admitting to yourself that you experience this emotion. Such admission is, as I discussed above, a necessary first step if you are to overcome your unhealthy envy. I will address this subject more fully in Chapter 5.

Another reason you may be reluctant to admit to yourself that you feel unhealthily envious is that, in your mind, such admission gives others the upper hand and puts you in a one-down position.

This is particularly the case with person-focused unhealthy envy, where you harbour malicious envy towards a friend and/ or family member whom you privately regard as worthier than yourself. Owning up to this belief is painful, and if you regard it as giving that person the upper hand over you, then you will be motivated to deny experiencing such feelings of unhealthy envy.

Refusing to take responsibility for your feelings of unhealthy envy

Just because you admit to yourself that you do experience feelings of unhealthy envy, it doesn't follow that you have taken responsibility for it. Thus, you may admit to feeling unhealthily envious, but blame your feelings on factors that are outside your control. For example, you may say, 'Yes, I do feel unhealthily envious, but that is because I was deprived of things as a child (or because I have inherited a tendency to think irrationally).' This has the effect of you having the sense that you are stuck with these feelings and that you can't do anything about them. Nothing is farther from the truth. You can do something about your feelings of unhealthy envy, if you accept the fact that they stem largely from a set of irrational beliefs and that you are responsible for holding these beliefs in the present. Yes, your childhood may be influential and you may even have a predisposition towards irrational thinking, but you feel unhealthily envious in the present because you are holding unhealthy envy-related irrational beliefs in the present. Those childhood or genetic factors just make it more likely that you will hold these beliefs, they don't make it inevitable that you will do so. Nor, more importantly, do they mean that you can't change these beliefs, although the presence of such factors may mean that you may have to work harder to change the beliefs than if they were absent.

This last issue points to another factor that may deter you

from taking responsibility for holding the irrational beliefs that underpin your feelings of unhealthy envy. Once you begin to see that your feelings of unhealthy envy are based on irrational beliefs that you have responsibility for holding, you will also see that to overcome these feelings you will need to change these irrational beliefs. In doing so, you may appreciate that changing irrational beliefs involves a fair measure of hard work, which you may not be prepared to do. To resolve this conflict you may think things over and deny that you have responsibility for your unhealthily envious feelings.

A final reason you may not take responsibility for your unhealthy envy and the irrational beliefs that underpin them involves self-depreciation. For you may think that if you are responsible for your feelings of unhealthy envy by holding a set of irrational beliefs, then this means that you are a stupid person for doing so. Rather than depreciating yourself in this way, you deny that you are responsible for largely creating your unhealthy envy. You admit to having these feelings, but you deny personal responsibility for them.

As I said earlier, I will show how you can take the first two steps to overcoming unhealthy envy, by admitting to having these feelings and taking personal responsibility for them, in Chapter 5. However, I have a number of issues to cover before getting to grips with helping you to overcome your unhealthy envy. First, I want to discuss a number of case histories of people who have experienced unhealthy envy of a friend or family member.

Case studies

In this section, I will discuss the cases of five people whose lives were affected for the worse by unhealthy envy. Four of the cases each exemplify one of the four major types of unhealthy envy that I discussed earlier: unhealthy object-focused ego envy, unhealthy object-focused non-ego envy, unhealthy person-focused ego envy and unhealthy person-focused non-ego envy. The fifth and final case exemplifies a mixed scenario. While these cases do not cover the entire range of problematic issues in unhealthy envy, they do give an adequate picture of the range of unhealthy envy-based problems.

To safeguard confidentiality, each 'case' is a composite of clients that I have seen over the years in my counselling practice. Each case is realistic in that it covers ground that is commonly encountered in unhealthy envy, but I have altered all identifiable material. This is now normal practice in writing up case histories for publication. We will meet our five 'cases' again in Chapter 6, when I show how they each overcame their unhealthy envy.

Before we meet the people behind the feeling, I want to remind you of a point that I made earlier in the chapter. The word 'object' in the phrase 'unhealthy object-focused envy' is used in a way that contrasts it with the term 'person' in 'unhealthy person-focused envy'. It points to *what* you envy rather than *who* you envy and it includes the following: material possessions; lifestyle (including wealth); personality characteristics; physical characteristics; relationships; social attention and/or recognition; public awards or honours; status and/or power.

Leonard: a case of unhealthy object-focused ego envy

Leonard is a 25-year-old single man who works as a messenger for a large city firm of solicitors. He considers himself to be a man's man, and likes going out with the lads and following Burnley FC, his favourite football team. Although he wouldn't put it in this way, Leonard has a 'macho' philosophy, where he values having a laugh with the lads, 'pulling birds', physical strength and emotional self-control. Unfortunately for Leonard, he has not been blessed with a physique to match his macho aspirations. Indeed, he is physically slight with poorly defined muscles. His friends tease him by calling him 'Skinny', which he hates, but he masks his feelings by laughing and joking in response to these teasing remarks.

Leonard experiences unhealthy object-focused ego envy about his male friends' muscular physique. His irrational belief that underpins his envy is as follows: 'I must be muscular like my male friends and because I am not I am a weed.'

As you can see, this belief is made up of a demand ('I must be muscular like my male friends') and a self-depreciation belief ('and because I am not I am a weed'). This shows that we are dealing with unhealthy ego envy. Also, Leonard's unhealthy envy with respect to his male friends is limited to bodily signs of masculinity, which shows that his unhealthy envy is object-focused.

When he held such a belief in situations where he was aware of his male friends' muscular frame in comparison to his own non-muscular frame, Leonard focused in his mind on the great unfairness of this state of affairs. He privately cursed his parents for being so puny themselves and tried to convince himself that being muscular wasn't important to him, when in reality it was. He also thought that all his male friends considered him to be a wimp, someone to kick around if he gave them the chance. These are the thinking consequences of his unhealthy envy-related ego irrational belief.

With respect to his behaviour, when he held the above irrational belief Leonard bought body-building magazines and sent away for body-building supplements. He would also go to the gym and work out for too long, with the result that he often had to seek physiotherapy for pulled muscles. In these ways he would jeopardize his health in order to improve his musculature.

Hilary: a case of unhealthy object-focused non-ego envy

Hilary is a 32-year-old married woman who is a solicitor. She has a good job, many friends and a husband who is devoted to her. They have been married for three years and plan to have children when Hilary is 35. Hilary has had a comfortable upbringing and has wanted for very little in her life.

Despite all of this, Hilary experiences unhealthy object-focused non-ego envy about her friends' possessions. Her irrational belief that underpins her envy is as follows: 'I must have the possessions that my friends have and that I don't have. If I don't then I can't bear the deprivation.'

As you can see, this belief is made up of a demand ('I must have the possessions that my friends have and that I don't have') and a low frustration tolerance belief ('If I don't then I can't bear the deprivation'). This shows that we are dealing with unhealthy non-ego envy. Also,

Hilary's unhealthy envy with respect to her friends is limited to material possessions but is not restricted to certain friends, which shows that her unhealthy envy is object-focused.

When she held such a belief in situations where she was aware that a friend had a possession that she did not have, Hilary dwelled on the deprivation that she 'felt'. This is all she could think about, and when in this frame of mind she could not acknowledge that her life was going well. The only thing that mattered to her was getting the possession that she was obsessed with. Thus, she would spend all of her time thinking how she could get what she believed was crucial to her happiness. At times when she despaired of ever getting what she believed she had to have in her life, Hilary even thought about how she could take the possession away from one of her friends or how she could spoil that person's enjoyment of it. These are the thinking consequences of her unhealthy envy-related non-ego irrational belief.

Behaviourally, Hilary translates some of her obsessive thoughts into action and often goes out to buy the said 'object'. In doing so, she gets herself ever deeper into debt, a fact that she tries to hide from her husband, family and friends. As a result, she sometimes engages in prostitution to fund her spending habits. She has also, at times, stolen the 'object' of her current desire, but to date she has not been caught. Invariably, when she finally gets the envied 'object' she experiences an initial rush of euphoria, followed by a vague sense of emptiness. As soon as she discovers that one of her friends has obtained something that she covets but does not have, she loses interest in the recently obtained 'object' and once again focuses on what she does not have. This pattern is frequently repeated. Although she thinks about how she can take the prized 'object' away from her friend or how she can spoil that person's enjoyment of it, she does not act on these thoughts, although she is very tempted to at times.

Jennifer: a case of unhealthy person-focused ego envy

Jennifer is a 23-year-old single woman who works in an office as an admin assistant. She has a small number of good friends and a larger number of acquaintances. Jennifer has a large number of brothers and sisters and a very large number of cousins, and was brought up by loving parents in a working-class area.

Jennifer's unhealthy envy is ego-based person-focused, in that she harbours envious feelings towards Barbara and Betty, two of her first cousins. She envies them many things, including their boyfriends, their relationship with one another, their looks and their clothes. In comparing herself to Barbara and Betty, Jennifer invariably feels badly about herself, which she covers up with her unhealthy envy-related thinking and behaviour. The irrational belief that underpins Jennifer's unhealthy envy is as follows: 'I must have what Barbara and Betty have. If I don't then this proves that I am inferior to them.'

As you can see, this belief is made up of a demand ('I must have what Barbara and Betty have') and a self-depreciation belief ('If I don't then I am inferior to them'). This shows that we are dealing with unhealthy non-ego envy. Also, Jennifer's unhealthy envy is limited to a few people and a large number of 'objects' that these people have that Jennifer considers she does not have, which shows that her unhealthy envy is person-focused.

When she held such a belief in situations where she was aware that Barbara and Betty had 'objects' that she did not have, Jennifer had an underlying feeling of shame about her envy and could not admit to herself or to others that she felt the way she did. Instead, she focused her attention on what she saw as Barbara and Betty's negative qualities as people. She told herself that they were arrogant, brash and bitchy. Instead of admitting that she found their boyfriends attractive and that she wished she could go out with such people, she put them down in her mind as being flash and chauvinistic.

Jennifer would also act on these negative thoughts, which were a product of her unhealthy envy-related irrational belief. For example, she took every opportunity to talk about Barbara and Betty in derogatory ways to the rest of her extended family and to her friends, and would even make up stories about them which put them in a negative light with her remaining family members. She wouldn't chat to Barbara and Betty, and when she had to talk to them she did not engage in eye contact with them and only gave them one-word answers to their questions. She would also, if she had the choice, avoid any family events attended by Barbara and Betty and when this wasn't possible she would spend the evening making bitchy remarks about them to others present. Things got so bad that her family stopped inviting her to large family events.

Tom: a case of unhealthy person-focused non-ego envy

Tom is a 43-year-old man who works as an insurance salesman. From schooldays, Tom has had a competitive relationship with Jim, a childhood friend whom he still sees regularly. Tom's parents were quite poor even though they lived in a prosperous community. This was due to the fact that Tom's mother inherited the family house from her mother. Given this, Tom was aware early on in his life that his contemporaries always had more than he did. He was not unduly bothered about this, but when it came to Jim it was a different matter. According to Tom, Jim was always bragging to Tom about what he had and made fun of Tom's poor background. Tom thought that this was unfair and was determined to prove that anything Jim could have, he could have.

Tom's unhealthy envy is non-ego-based and person-focused in that he harbours envious feelings towards a given person, his friend Jim. However, Tom does not think that he is inferior if he does not have what Jim has. Rather, he focuses on the deprivation he experiences, which he believes he cannot bear. The irrational belief that underpins Tom's unhealthy envy is as follows: 'I must have what Jim has. I can't bear being deprived in this way.'

As you can see, this belief is made up of a demand ('I must have what Jim has') and a low frustration tolerance ('I can't bear being deprived in this way'). This shows that we are dealing with unhealthy non-ego envy. Also, Tom's' unhealthy envy is limited to one person, Jim, and a large number of material possessions that Jim has that Tom does not have, which shows that his unhealthy envy is person-focused.

When Tom held such a belief in situations where he was aware that Jim had possessions that he did not have, he spent a lot of time thinking about how he could get what Jim had and he lacked. He also considered it to be grossly unfair that Jim had the wherewithal to have so many possessions without having to work hard for them, while he, Tom, worked his fingers to the bone and yet had little money for the luxuries in life that seemed to be there for the taking for Jim. In this respect, it is worth noting that Jim's family were very rich and Jim had in his teens inherited a lot of money, with the effect that he did not have to work hard for a living.

Behaviourally, Tom's unhealthy envy-related irrational belief led him to go into debt in his attempts to get what he believed he must not be deprived of – goods that Jim had recently bought and bragged about and which he, Tom, did not have. Tom had recently borrowed a large sum of money from a loan shark to fund his profligate spending, since he had exceeded the limits on each of his three credit cards.

He also spent a large amount of time complaining to anyone who would listen about the unfairness of a system that allowed spongers like Jim to thrive without hard work, while others worked hard for little gain. Gradually, Tom had alienated his friends and family and had taken to drink to console himself now that there was nobody to listen to his woes.

Samantha: a case of mixed unhealthy envy

So far, I have presented case studies of people whose unhealthy envy was fairly pure. In other words, the individual's unhealthy envy was either person-focused or object-focused and either ego or non-ego in nature. I chose to present these 'pure types' to help you clearly understand the processes involved. However, in reality, much unhealthy envy is mixed in nature rather than pure. This is shown in the case of Samantha.

Samantha is a 45-year-old unmarried woman who works as a hardware consultant in IT. She lives alone and has few friends. She is very bright, but is quite lazy and has never fulfilled her intellectual potential. She experiences much unhealthy envy in her life. In terms of person-focused envy she envies her two sisters, who are more attractive, more successful and more popular than she is, and who are both happily married with loving husbands and well-adjusted children. Samantha's unhealthy person-focused envy is both ego and non-ego in nature. From an ego perspective, she holds the following irrational belief which comprises a demand and a self-depreciation belief: 'I must have what my sisters have and if I don't then it proves that I am inferior to them as a person.'

When Samantha believes this, she then focuses on all of her perceived inadequacies and edits out her strengths. In this frame of mind she used to phone the few friends she had and complain endlessly to them about how worthless she is. An initial sympathetic and reassuring response from these friends turned to exasperation, hostility and avoidance when Samantha's self-depreciating telephone calls became increasingly regular. In the absence of anybody to talk to, Samantha has increasingly turned to food and drink to cope with her feelings of unhealthy envy and depression. This compounds the problem because she is now overweight and alcohol exacerbates her lethargy and inactivity, meaning that she achieves less and less while her sisters are achieving more and more. This only serves to lead Samantha to feel increasing unhealthy envy via the above-mentioned irrational belief.

From a non-ego perspective, Samantha's person-focused unhealthy envy is based on the following irrational belief, which comprises a demand and an awfulizing belief: 'It's unfair that my sisters have what I don't have and want, and it absolutely should not be this way. It's truly awful that this unfairness exists.'

When she holds this belief, Samantha's frame of mind is dominated by thoughts of all the unfairnesses she has experienced in life that have involved her sisters. Because she has nobody to talk to she has taken to telephoning the Samaritans when she is in this mindset, and she spends hours talking to people whose role it is to give a listening, non-judgemental response. Samantha has recently become heavily reliant on phoning the Samaritans whenever she is in a self-pitying mood dominated by unhealthy envy. The response that she gets from their volunteers seems to reinforce her self-pity.

In addition to her person-focused unhealthy envy, Samantha also experiences object-focused unhealthy envy. In particular, she harbours unhealthily envious feelings towards her friends who are successful in their careers. In this respect her ego-based object-focused unhealthy envy stems from the following irrational belief, which comprises a demand and a self-depreciation belief: 'I must be as successful in my career as my friends are in theirs, and if I'm not then it proves that I am inadequate.'

In the wake of this irrational belief, Samantha thought that she did not have what it takes to be successful in her own career, and consequently she did not think about ways that she could better her own career prospects. Behaviourally, therefore, she refused her manager's offers to sponsor her to go on training seminars and made no attempt to keep up to date with developments in her field. The consequence of this was that she made it unlikely that her organization would promote her and this, in her mind, reinforced her own sense of personal inadequacy.

Samantha's object-focused unhealthy envy was also non-ego in nature. Here, she focused on the benefits her friends derived from being successful in their careers that she lacked by not being successful in hers. The irrational belief that underpinned this type of unhealthy envy was comprised of a demand and a low frustration tolerance belief, as follows: 'I must have the benefits that my friends who are successful in their careers have, and it is unbearable that I don't.'

When under the influence of this irrational belief, Samantha daydreamed of having these benefits, but whenever she reminded herself of the reality of her deprivation she felt sorry for herself for not having what others have. Behaviourally, she ate and drank to deal with the pain of her unhealthy envy-influenced deprivation.

We will return to the cases of Leonard, Hilary, Jennifer, Tom and Samantha in Chapter 6, where I will discuss how each of them overcame their feelings of unhealthy envy. Meanwhile, in the next chapter I will help you to understand the nature of healthy envy.

3

The ABCs of healthy envy

Introduction

As I have discussed in a number of my self-help books for Sheldon Press, one of the problems with the English language is that it does not have suitable words for healthy negative emotions, i.e. emotions that are negative to experience but represent constructive responses to negative life events. Given this fact, and as previously discussed in Chapter 1, I refer to unhealthy envy to denote envy when it is negative and unhealthy, and healthy envy to denote envy which is negative but healthy. For envy can be healthy, and in this chapter I will focus on healthy envy and factors associated with it. This is important, since in certain situations it is appropriate for you to feel healthily envious and much of what I have to say in this book will be to encourage you to overcome unhealthy envy and to feel healthy envy instead.

In this chapter, then, I will consider what people tend to be healthily envious about and discuss the rational beliefs that underpin healthy envy. I will also consider what people tend to do and think when they experience healthy envy. I will again use the ABC framework discussed in Chapter 1 to structure the material.

Common features between healthy envy and unhealthy envy

Healthy envy and unhealthy envy are similar in four main respects. They have the same theme and the same components that comprise this theme, they are about the same things, and they can be both object-focused and person-focused. Let me elaborate.

Healthy envy and unhealthy envy share the same theme and the same components

As I pointed out in Chapter 2, this key theme is as follows:

> You feel envious (healthily or unhealthily) about someone else having that which you prize but which you do not possess.

If we break this theme down into its component parts, we have:

- You.
- Someone else. (This can be one person or a group of people. It can be a racial group, a national group or a religious group.)
- Something that you prize. (Again, as you will see, this can be quite varied.)
- The other possesses what you prize and do not have: this is the central component of all envy, both healthy and unhealthy.

As I noted above, what you envy can be very varied and depends very much on your idiosyncratic desires. Without attempting to be comprehensive, let me list some of the major things that you may envy that a family member or friend has that you do not possess. Remember, this is the same for both healthy and unhealthy envy.

- A material possession or possessions
- Lifestyle (including wealth)
- A personality characteristic
- A physical characteristic
- A relationship or relationships
- Social attention and/or recognition
- Public awards or honours
- Status and/or power.

Healthy envy (and unhealthy envy) can be both object-focused and person-focused

Both types of envy, healthy and unhealthy, can be largely object-focused or person-focused. Here, I will highlight healthy envy.

Object-focused healthy envy

When your healthy envy is object-focused your focus is on the 'object' (a generic term that I have given to all the items listed above) that another has and you don't have, rather than on the person who has it. In this type of envy you don't even have to know the other person to feel healthy envy about what he or she has, although as this book is about envy in friendships and families you will know that person. An example of object-focused healthy envy is when you feel healthily envious on seeing that a friend has a new sports car and your envy is focused on the car rather than the person who has the car. This type of envy is called object-focused envy because *what* you envy is more relevant than *who* you envy.

Person-focused healthy envy

When your healthy envy is person-focused, who you envy is more relevant than what you envy. While the content of the healthy and unhealthy object-focused envy is the same (for instance, you can feel healthily or unhealthily envious about the same sports car), who you envy in healthy person-focused envy and unhealthy person-focused envy can be the same or it can be very different. In this section, I will concentrate on situations when who you envy in both types is the same, and in the next section I will discuss occasions when they are very different.

When you are unhealthily envious of a friend or family member you tend to have a competitive relationship with that person and, as I discussed in Chapter 2, you tend to 'feel' inferior to the person, although you find this hard to acknowledge to yourself. It is possible to have a competitive relationship with a friend or family member, but to manage that relationship well in that you don't 'feel' inferior to that person.

How healthy envy differs from unhealthy envy

While healthy envy shares some of the features of unhealthy envy, it has more differences than similarities. In this section, I will focus on how healthy envy differs from unhealthy envy. If you read it carefully, you will have good understanding of healthy envy.

Person-focused healthy envy differs from its unhealthy counterpart

In Chapter 2, I discussed the nature of person-focused unhealthy envy and emphasized that when you harbour feelings of unhealthy envy towards a friend or family member, that person is generally speaking someone (1) to whom you consider yourself to be inferior and/or (2) with whom you consider yourself to be in unhealthy competition (in the sense that you believe that you *have to* beat or equal that person). I showed above that it is possible to have such a relationship and feel healthily envious of the person as long as you don't 'feel' inferior to that person.

In addition, and this does not occur in unhealthy envy, when your person-focused envy is healthy, that friend or family member can also be someone whom you admire and would like to emulate: in other words, someone who tends to serve as a role model for you. You don't 'feel' inferior to the person and you don't tend have an unhealthily competitive relationship with him or her in the sense that you think that you have to beat or equal them.

In person-focused healthy envy, when you do envy 'objects'

it is usually because the friend or family member whom you admire has them. If another person had those same 'objects' you probably would not prize them.

Why your feelings of healthy envy are very different from your feelings of unhealthy envy

The main difference between healthy envy and unhealthy envy lies in the different beliefs that underpin these different emotions. Let me make this clear by using the ABC example that I first discussed in Chapter 2. If you recall, in that example I asked you to suppose that you and a friend went for the same job and that he got the job. Using the situational ABC framework, if your envy was unhealthy in nature we would have the following:

Situation = My friend and I both went for a job, which he got.
'A' = He has the job that I wanted but didn't get.
'B' = Irrational beliefs.
'C' = Unhealthy envy.

If your envy were healthy, however, the situational ABC would be as follows:

Situation = My friend and I both went for a job, which he got.
'A' = He has the job that I wanted but didn't get.
'B' = Rational beliefs.
'C' = Healthy envy.

To reiterate what I said in Chapter 2, according to REBT theory, while your emotions are influenced by situations and in particular the inferences that you make about these situations (at 'A'), neither these situations nor the inferences at 'A' determine your emotions. Rather, it is the beliefs that you hold about these situations and in particular about the inferences that you form about the situations that have a much greater determining effect on the way that you feel (and the way that you act and subsequently think, for that matter). The two examples that I have just presented show that if you hold a set of rational beliefs (at 'B') about someone getting a job that you wanted but didn't get (at 'A'), then your feelings of envy (at 'C') will be healthy. However, if your beliefs are irrational in the same set of circumstances, then your feelings of envy will be unhealthy.

In Chapter 2, I examined this scenario in detail, having assumed that the person's envy was unhealthy and thereby based on irrational beliefs. In this chapter I will examine the scenario assuming this time that the person's envy was healthy in nature and thereby based on rational beliefs. I will now discuss these rational beliefs in the context of four types of healthy envy. These are:

- healthy ego envy: object-focused
- healthy non-ego envy: object-focused
- healthy ego envy: person-focused
- healthy non-ego envy: person-focused.

While in practice your healthy envy may have elements of one or more of these different types, I will here consider them in their pure form.

Healthy ego envy: object-focused

In this type of healthy envy, your focus is on the job that your friend got and that you wanted but didn't get. Since your healthy envy is ego in nature, your rational beliefs reflect this as in the following:

Situation = My friend and I both went for a job, which he got.
'A' = Not having *a job* like the one my friend got.
'B' = (1) I would like to have *a job* like the one he has, but I do not absolutely have to have one. (Non-dogmatic preference)
(2) I am not less worthy because I don't have *a job* like the one he has. My worth as a person is fixed and isn't affected by whether or not I have such *a job*. (Self-acceptance belief)
'C' = Healthy envy.

Note the following in the above ABC analysis:

1 In 'A', the emphasis is on the job and not on the person who has the job. It is likely, therefore, that you may have felt healthily envious if other people had got the job and you hadn't.

2 I have concentrated on your non-dogmatic preference and self-acceptance belief since these are the most salient in healthy object-focused ego envy.

Healthy non-ego envy: object-focused

In this type of healthy envy, your focus is again on the job that your friend got and that you wanted, but didn't get. Since your healthy envy is non-ego in nature, your rational beliefs reflect this, as in the following:

> Situation = My friend and I both went for a job, which he got.
> 'A' = Not having *a job* like the one my friend got.
> 'B' = (1) I would like to have *a job* like the one he has, but I do not absolutely have to have one. (Non-dogmatic preference)
> (2) It's bad, but not the end of the world, that I don't have *a job* like the one my friend got. (Non-awfulizing belief)
> (3) I can bear being deprived of what I want, i.e. a job like the one he got, although it is difficult to do so. (High frustration tolerance belief)
> 'C' = Healthy envy.

Note the following in the above ABC analysis:

1 In 'A' the emphasis is again on the job and not on the person who has the job. It is again likely that you may have felt healthily envious if other people had got the job and you hadn't.

2 I have concentrated on your non-dogmatic preference, non-awfulizing and HFT beliefs, since these are the most salient in healthy object-focused non-ego envy. However, in future when I discuss healthy non-ego envy I will feature the non-dogmatic preference and either the non-awfulizing belief or

an HFT belief, since one of these latter two beliefs (together with the non-dogmatic preference) is usually sufficient to account for this type of healthy envy.

Healthy ego envy: person-focused

In this type of healthy envy, your focus is on your friend who got the job rather than on the job itself. Since your healthy envy is ego in nature, your rational beliefs reflect this, as in the following:

> Situation = My friend and I both went for a job, which he got.
> 'A' = *My friend* having something (a job) that I don't have, but want.
> 'B' = (1) I would like to have what *he* has, but I don't have to have it. (Non-dogmatic preference)
> (2) I am not less worthy than *he* is, even though I don't have what he has. I am an unrateable, fallible human being who hasn't got what I would like. (Self-acceptance belief)
> 'C' = Healthy envy.

Note the following in the above ABC analysis:

1 In 'A', the emphasis is on your friend and not on the job. It is likely, therefore, that you may feel healthily envious towards this person for other things that he may have that you lack, whereas you may not feel unhealthily envious towards another person who has what you don't have but desire.

2 I have once again concentrated on your non-dogmatic preference and self-acceptance belief, since these are the most salient in healthy, person-focused ego envy.

Healthy non-ego envy: person-focused

In this type of healthy envy, your focus is once again on your friend and not on the job. Since your healthy envy is non-ego in nature, your rational beliefs reflect this, as in the following:

Situation = My friend and I both went for a job, which he got.
Critical 'A' = It is unfair that *he* got the job that I wanted but didn't get.
'B' = (1) It is undesirable that this unfairness – where *my friend* got what I wanted – exists, but there is no reason why this situation must be fair. (Non-dogmatic preference)
(2) It is bad, but not terrible, that this unfairness – where *he* got what I wanted – has occurred. (Non-awfulizing belief)
'C' = Healthy envy.

Note the following in the above ABC analysis:

1 In 'A', the emphasis is on the unfairness that your friend got the job rather than on the unfairness that you didn't get the job. It is likely that you will feel healthily envious if this named person experiences other unfair (as deemed by you) advantages.

2 I have concentrated on your non-dogmatic preference and non-awfulizing belief here. I could also have focused on your non-dogmatic preference and HFT belief.

The differences in how you subsequently think when you hold a healthy envy-related rational belief compared to when you hold an unhealthy envy-related irrational belief

When you hold a set of healthy envy-related rational beliefs, these beliefs will influence how you subsequently think. These thoughts tend to be elaborations on the healthy envy theme, and/or relevant inferences and/or action-related, and are different from thoughts that are influenced by your unhealthy envy-related irrational beliefs. While the thinking that stems from your unhealthy envy-related irrational belief takes a variety of different forms, much of it distorted (see Chapter 2), the thinking that stems from holding a healthy envy-related rational belief is far less varied and is characterized by realism (as shown below).

Thinking about how to get what you envy only if it is useful to you, it is attainable and if pursuing it is not too costly

When you are healthily envious and you desire, but do not demand, that you must get what your friend or family member has that you lack, then you will tend to think about whatever it is that you covet, but don't have. Your thoughts will not only concern the 'object', but also how to get it. When your thoughts are in this direction, you tend to think of the usefulness of the 'object' to you, whether or not it is attainable, and the price that you may have to pay (financially and psychologically) in your pursuit of the 'object'. If it isn't really useful to you, if it isn't attainable or if the price of pursuing it is too great, then you will tend to stop thinking of ways of getting it. Compare this to the thinking that you engage in when under the influence of your unhealthy envy-related irrational belief, where, as I discussed in Chapter 2, you think of ways of getting the coveted 'object' regardless of its true usefulness to you, its attainability or the price that you may have to pay in pursuing it.

What you don't think when you hold healthy envy-related rational beliefs

As I discussed above, the main type of thinking that you engage in when you hold a healthy envy-related rational belief concerns satisfying yourself that you really want what you covet, that it is useful to you, that you can attain it and that the costs of pursuing it are manageable. Given this, the thinking that you engage in once you hold a healthy envy-related rational belief differs from that which stems from holding an unhealthy envy-related irrational belief in what you *don't* think. Thus:

1 You tend not to think about depriving your friend or family member of what you envy. Rather, your thoughts are focused

on the good points of the 'object' of your envy and how you can get it.

2 You tend to accept not having what you want and don't think that it is unfair to be deprived unless it is objectively unfair.

3 You tend not to think about spoiling or destroying what you covet so that your friend or family member does not have it. Again, your thoughts are focused on the good aspects of what you covet and how you can get it.

4 You tend not to think denigrating thoughts about what you envy. Rather, your thoughts are positive about it.

5 You tend not to think denigrating thoughts about who you envy even if you are in competition with the friend or family member. Again, your thoughts are positive about what you envy about the friend or family member, even if the person is a rival.

6 You tend not to try to convince yourself that you are happy with what you have. Rather, you acknowledge to yourself that you do want what you covet and are not defensive about this.

7 The thinking you engage in that stems from a healthy envy-related rational belief tends not to be obsessive.

The differences in your behaviour when you hold a healthy envy-related rational belief compared to when you hold an unhealthy envy-related irrational belief

So far I have considered:

• what you make yourself healthily envious about (usually someone having something that you want but don't have, where the focus is either on the 'object' itself or on the friend or family member who happens to have the 'object');

- how you make yourself healthily envious (by holding one or more rational beliefs about the above situation);
- the thinking consequences of holding these healthy envy-based rational beliefs.

In this section, I will consider the behavioural consequences of holding healthy envy-related rational beliefs and compare them with the behavioural consequences of holding unhealthy envy-related irrational beliefs. Before I do so, I want to reiterate one point that I made when discussing the behavioural consequences of holding unhealthy envy-related irrational beliefs.

- Healthy envy-related behavioural consequences are frequently the behavioural expressions of the thinking consequences of holding healthy envy-related rational beliefs. In this way, thinking and behaviour often go together.

When you hold a set of healthy envy-related rational beliefs, you then act or tend to act in one or more of the following ways:

How you do act when you hold envy-related rational beliefs

Seeking out what you envy when you truly want it, when you can achieve it and when the costs of doing so are not prohibitive is the main behavioural consequence of holding a healthy envy-related rational belief, and is the behavioural expression of the major thinking consequence of holding such a belief. This is in direct contrast to how you act (or 'feel' like acting) when you hold an unhealthy envy-related irrational belief, i.e. pursuing what you covet irrespective of whether it is attainable or useful to you, or irrespective of the costs involved in doing so, or not pursuing it because you don't think that you can get it.

How you don't act when you hold healthy envy-related rational beliefs

The main type of thinking and acting that you engage in when you hold a healthy envy-related rational belief concerns first satisfying yourself that you really want what you covet, that it is useful to you, that you can attain it and that the costs of pursuing it are manageable, and then acting in ways that are consistent with such realistic judgements. Given this, the behaviour that you engage in once you hold a healthy envy-related rational belief differs from that which stems from holding an unhealthy envy-related irrational belief in how you *don't* act. Thus, when you hold a healthy envy-related rational belief:

1 You do not cast aside what you covet once you have got it. Rather, you keep it and make appropriate use of it.
2 You do not attempt to take away what you covet from your friend or family member. You are quite prepared for that person to have and enjoy what he or she has.
3 You do not strive to spoil or destroy someone else's coveted 'object'. Again, you are quite prepared for that person to have and enjoy what he or she has.
4 You neither verbally disparage the friend or family member whom you healthily envy to others, nor encourage others to disparage the person. Rather, you are complimentary about your friend or family member and tell other people what you envy about him or her.
5 You neither verbally disparage the 'object' that you healthily envy to others, nor encourage them to disparage the 'object'. Rather, you are complimentary about the 'object' and tell others what you like about it and why you want it.
6 In your dealings with others you do not deny that you feel healthily envious. This is because you tend not to feel ashamed of these healthy but negative feelings, unlike the shame that you would tend to experience about your unhealthy envy. Rather, you are open and honest about your feelings to yourself and to others.

Having discussed the nature of both unhealthy and healthy

envy, I will now turn my attention to showing you how to overcome your feelings of unhealthy envy. In the next chapter, then, I will discuss how you can deal with specific episodes of unhealthy envy.

4

How to deal with specific episodes of unhealthy envy

Introduction

Whether you are prone to unhealthy envy or you only experience this destructive emotion in given situations, it is important that you begin the change process by dealing with specific episodes of unhealthy envy.

I will now present a 13-step guide to overcoming situationally based unhealthy envy.

> In taking you through these steps I will use the experience of Dorothy, a client of mine who chose a specific example of object-focused non-ego unhealthy envy for consideration. While the work that I did with her occurred within a counselling context, the blueprint is the same whether you are seeing a counsellor or whether you are using this material on your own.
>
> Basically, Dorothy was unhealthily envious about a friend being promoted to a position at work that she herself coveted, but did not have.

Step 1: Acknowledge that you felt unhealthy envy in the situation to be analysed and that this emotion is unhealthy

In order to overcome situationally based unhealthy envy, it is important that you select a situation in which you experience unhealthy envy. If you choose a situation in which you experienced healthy envy you will be trying to change an emotion that is healthy, and if you do this then this 13-step sequence won't work. So, it is important that you distinguish between healthy and unhealthy envy. There are two major ways of doing so.

First, you need to identify how you thought when you felt envious. If your envy was unhealthy, your subsequent thinking would have probably been along some or all of the following lines:

- You tend to think about how to get what you envy regardless of its usefulness, its attainability and the cost of pursuing it.
- You tend to think about depriving your friend or family member of what he or she has that you envy.
- You tend to think that not having what you want is unfair whether it is unfair or not.
- You tend to think about spoiling or destroying what you covet so that your friend or family member does not have it.
- You tend to think denigrating thoughts about what you envy.
- You tend to think denigrating thoughts about the person you envy.
- You tend to convince yourself that you are happy with what you have.
- The thinking consequences of holding unhealthy envy-based irrational beliefs can be obsessive.

However, if your envy was healthy your subsequent thinking would have been characterized by some or all of the following:

- You tend to think about how to get what you envy only if it is useful to you, if it is attainable and if pursuing it is not too costly.
- You tend not to think about depriving your friend or family member of what he or she has that you envy. Rather, your thoughts are focused on the good points of what you envy and how you can get it.

- You tend to accept not having what you want and don't think that it is unfair to be deprived unless it is objectively unfair.
- You tend not to think about spoiling or destroying what you covet so that your friend or family member does not have it. Again, your thoughts are focused on the good aspects of what you covet and how you can get it.
- You tend not to think denigrating thoughts about what you covet. Rather, your thoughts are positive about it.
- You tend not to think denigrating thoughts about the person you envy even if you are in competition with that friend or family member. Again, your thoughts are basically realistic about the envied friend or family member.
- You tend not to try to convince yourself that you are happy with what you have. Rather, you acknowledge to yourself that you do want what you covet and are not defensive about this.
- The thinking you engage in that stems from a healthy envy-related rational belief tends not to be obsessive.

Second, you need to identify how you acted (or 'felt' like acting) when you experienced your feelings of envy. If your envy was unhealthy, you would have acted (or 'felt' like acting) in one or more of the following ways:

- You pursue what you covet irrespective of whether it is attainable or useful to you and regardless of the costs involved. When you get the prized 'object' you will tend to discard it fairly quickly.
- You actively attempt to take away what you covet from your friend or family member.
- You actively strive to spoil or destroy your friend's or family member's coveted 'object'.
- You verbally disparage to others the friend or family member whom you unhealthily envy, and encouraging them to disparage the person.
- You verbally disparage to others the 'object' that you

unhealthily envy and encourage them to disparage the 'object'.

- You tell others that you don't really want what you do, in truth, covet.

However, if your envy was healthy, you acted (or 'felt' like acting) in one or more of the following ways:

- You seek out what you envy when you truly want it, when you can achieve it and when the costs of doing so are not prohibitive.
- You do not cast aside what you envy once you have got it. Rather, you keep it and make appropriate use of it.
- You do not attempt to take away what you covet from your friend or family member. You are quite prepared for this person to have and enjoy what he or she has.
- You do not strive to spoil or destroy your friend's or family member's coveted 'object'. Again, you are quite prepared for this person to have and enjoy what he or she has.
- You do not verbally disparage to others your friend's or family member whom you healthily envy, nor encourage these others to disparage the person. Rather, you are complimentary about your friend or family member and tell other people what you envy about him or her.
- You do not verbally disparage to others the 'object' that you healthily envy, nor encourage them to disparage the 'object'. Rather, you are complimentary about the 'object' and tell other people what you like about it and why you want it.

Dorothy acknowledged that her envy was unhealthy. She realized that her increasing preoccupation about the unfairness of being passed over for the position that she coveted, and the fact that she was beginning to plan how to sabotage her friend when she took up the coveted job, indicated that her envy was unhealthy.

Step 2: Choose a specific example of your unhealthy envy and be as concrete as possible

Once you have decided that your envy is unhealthy, the next step is for you to choose a specific example of it. Guard against a tendency, which many people have, to think of your unhealthy envy in vague terms. Doing so will make it difficult for you to get information that is specific enough to help you to identify the specific irrational beliefs that underpin your feelings of unhealthy envy.

Choosing a specific example of your unhealthy envy and being as concrete about it as you can will enable you to identify your specific unhealthy envy-based irrational beliefs.

> Dorothy's initial account of her unhealthy envy problem already referred to a specific example of this problem. If you recall, it was that she was unhealthily envious about a friend being promoted to a position at work that she coveted, but did not have.

Step 3: Acknowledge that healthy envy is the constructive alternative to unhealthy envy

In order to change your feelings of unhealthy envy, it is important that you have a clear idea of what to change them to. In the preceding chapter, I pointed out that healthy envy is the constructive alternative to unhealthy envy and discussed its main features. Thus, if you are aware that someone has something you covet, but do not have, it is important that you see that healthy envy is a healthy emotional response to this situation. It would not be healthy for you to be indifferent about this situation, for example, because this would involve you lying to yourself and trying to persuade yourself that it didn't matter to you whether you had what you covet or not. Since lying to yourself is not a constructive way of dealing with emotional problems, I encourage you to see the value of healthy envy and suggest that you reread Chapter 3 if you are unsure about this.

> Once the concept of healthy envy was explained to Dorothy, she could see that she could feel badly but healthily about not getting what she coveted and that this meant that she could concentrate on other aspects of her life. She accepted that, in this case, healthy envy was a constructive and viable alternative to the unhealthy envy that she experienced.

Step 4: Accept yourself for feeling unhealthy envy

Before you begin to analyse the concrete example that you have selected in Step 2, it is important that you ask yourself the following question: 'Did I depreciate myself in any significant way for experiencing unhealthy envy?' If the answer is yes, you are in good company: research has shown that unhealthy envy is one of the most frequently cited emotions that people feel ashamed about experiencing, and this shame often leads them to deny that they experience this emotion when in reality they do.

If you did depreciate yourself for feeling unhealthy envy, it is important that you deal with this issue before proceeding further with your chosen example of unhealthy envy. If you try to bypass your feelings of self-depreciation about feeling unhealthily envious, these self-depreciation-based feelings will interfere with you working to overcome your unhealthy envy.

What do you need to do if you did depreciate yourself? First, it is important that you acknowledge that while unhealthy envy is a destructive emotion it is a common one and many people experience it. It is part of the human condition and no human is beyond experiencing it. That doesn't mean that it is healthy, though, but it is common. While it is a destructive emotion, you are not an abnormal human being for experiencing it. Rather, you are a fallible human being for experiencing this emotion even though it is, as I have just said, unhealthy.

Second, even if you think of your unhealthy envy as a loathsome emotion, this does not mean that you are a loathsome person. Your feelings of unhealthy envy are only a part of you and cannot define you. In reality, you are a complex, imperfect person with an envy problem and it is important that you remind yourself of this fact as you work on overcoming it.

Third, when you depreciate yourself for feeling unhealthy envy, you are demanding that you must not feel this way in the first place. However, the truth is that you did experience unhealthy envy. If there was a law of the universe to prevent you from feeling unhealthy envy, then you would not have experienced this feeling in the first place, nor could you have done so. But we know that the reality was that you did experience such feelings, which proves that there is no such law. Remind yourself of this next time you find yourself depreciating yourself for feeling unhealthy envy.

Accepting yourself for feeling unhealthy envy when you do so will help you to address the issues that led you to feel this way in the first place, so that you can work towards experiencing healthy envy instead.

Dorothy initially felt ashamed about her feelings of unhealthy envy because she believed that her feelings proved she was a terrible person. She could see that these feelings of shame posed a barrier to addressing the factors that led to her feelings of unhealthy envy. I helped her to see that while her feelings might be unedifying, this did not prove that she was a terrible person – rather, she was an ordinary person capable of healthy and unhealthy responses to events. She accepted this and felt disappointed instead of ashamed, which helped her to concentrate on the factors that needed to be taken into account if she was to overcome her unhealthy envy.

Step 5: Identify your 'A' and assume temporarily that this 'A' is true

You are now in a position to identify what you felt most unhealthily envious about in the specific episode under consideration. From what I have already written, you will know that you are unhealthily envious about someone else having that which you prize but which you do not possess. As I discussed in Chapter 2, the focus of your unhealthy envy can be on your friend or family member (i.e. you envy the person rather than what the person has) or on the 'object' that your friend or family member has (i.e. you envy what the person has rather than the person).

> Dorothy identified her 'A' as 'my friend getting the position that I coveted and deserved to get'.

After you have identified your 'A', it is very important for you to treat it as though it were true, at least for the time being. The reason for this is that doing so allows you to identify the irrational beliefs that are at the core of your feelings of unhealthy envy.

> If, at this stage, Dorothy had challenged her inference that not getting the coveted position was unfair, she would have deprived herself of dealing with the real determinant of her unhealthy envy: her irrational beliefs.

So, to reiterate, at this point resist any temptation you may experience to reinterpret your 'A'. There will be a better opportunity for you to do so later, after you have modified the irrational beliefs that are at the core of your feelings of unhealthy envy.

Step 6: Understand that your feelings of unhealthy envy stem largely from your irrational beliefs about this lack and are not caused by the lack itself

Throughout this book I have emphasized that activating events, or 'A's to be more precise, contribute to but do not cause your feelings, behaviour and subsequent thinking at point 'C' in the ABC framework. Rather, how you feel, act and think depends largely (but not exclusively) on the beliefs that you hold about these 'A's.

> Once I had explained REBT's ABC model of unhealthy envy, Dorothy fully accepted that her feelings of unhealthy envy were largely determined by her irrational beliefs.

Step 7: Identify your irrational beliefs and discriminate them from their rational alternatives

After you have fully accepted the view that your feelings of unhealthy envy are largely determined by your irrational beliefs, the next step is to identify the specific irrational beliefs that you held in the specific episode under consideration. In doing so, it is important that you distinguish these irrational beliefs from their rational alternatives. This task is fairly straightforward if you bear in mind the points that I made in Chapters 2 and 3. You will recall that there are four major irrational beliefs:

- rigid demands
- awfulizing beliefs
- low frustration tolerance beliefs
- depreciation beliefs.

The rational alternatives to these irrational beliefs are as follows:

- non-dogmatic preferences
- non-awfulizing beliefs

- high frustration tolerance beliefs
- acceptance beliefs.

> Dorothy identified her irrational belief as follows: 'My friend
> absolutely should not have got the position that I coveted and
> deserved to get but didn't. I absolutely should have got it myself and
> it is awful that she got it and I didn't.' She was able to discriminate
> this from her potential rational belief: 'I would have much preferred it
> if my friend had not got the position that I coveted and deserved to
> get and that I had got it myself, but sadly there is no reason why this
> had to occur, and while it is bad that it didn't, it isn't awful.'

Step 8: Challenge these irrational beliefs by showing yourself that they are false, illogical and self-defeating

Now that you have identified the specific irrational beliefs that underpin your feelings of unhealthy envy, the next step is for you to challenge these beliefs. The purpose of challenging is to understand fully why your irrational belief is irrational and thus to begin to undermine your conviction in it. You do this by asking yourself and answering three questions:

- Is my irrational belief helpful or unhelpful? Does it give me healthy or unhealthy results?
- Is my irrational belief true or false? Is it consistent or inconsistent with reality?
- Is my irrational belief sensible or nonsensical? Is it logical or illogical?

> This is how Dorothy challenged her irrational belief (comprised of a
> rigid demand and an awfulizing belief): 'My friend absolutely should
> not have got the position that I coveted and deserved to get but
> didn't. I absolutely should have got it myself and it is awful that she
> got it and I didn't.'
>
> *Question:* Is this belief helpful or unhelpful?

Answer: It is unhelpful. As long as I demand that she absolutely should not have got the position and that I should have done so, I am going to feel unhealthy envy and this is going to do nothing to reverse the situation. The same is the case for the belief that it is awful that she got the position and I didn't.

Question: Is this belief true or false?
Answer: It is false. If there was a law of the universe that decreed that I absolutely should have got the position and that she absolutely shouldn't have, then this what would have had to have happened. As it didn't my demand is false. Also, if it were true that her getting the position rather than me was awful, then nothing could be worse. I can think of plenty of things that could have been worse than this.

Question: Is this belief logical or illogical?
Answer: It is illogical. If we take my demand we can see that it has two components: an asserted preference component and an asserted demand component. Thus: 'Because it would have been desirable for me to get the position rather than her (asserted preference component) therefore it absolutely should have been that way (asserted demand component).' My asserted preference that it would have been desirable if I had got the position rather than her is not rigid, but the asserted demand component that it absolutely should have been that way is rigid. Logically you cannot derive something rigid from something non-rigid, and therefore my demand is illogical.

If we take my awfulizing belief, we can see that it also has two components: an asserted badness component and an asserted awfulizing component. Thus: 'Because it would be bad if she got the position and I didn't (asserted badness component), therefore it is awful (asserted awfulizing component).' My asserted badness component that it would be bad if she got the position rather than me is non-extreme and the asserted awfulizing component is extreme. Therefore my awfulizing belief is illogical because logically you cannot derive something extreme from something non-extreme.

Using the same questions, query the irrational belief that underpins your situationally based unhealthy envy. The more you challenge the irrational beliefs and really see that they are unhelpful, false and illogical, the more you will be motivated to gain conviction in their rational alternatives.

Step 9: Show yourself that the rational alternatives to these irrational beliefs, by contrast, are true, sensible and yield healthy results

When you challenge your irrational beliefs it is akin to uprooting the weeds in a garden. However, if you want flowers in your garden you will also have to prepare the ground and plant seeds so that these flowers will grow and flourish. Thus, if your rational beliefs are to grow and flourish, you will have to sow them into your belief system.

The first step in this process is to ask and answer the same questions that you posed of your irrational beliefs in the previous step. Doing so enables you to see clearly why your rational belief is rational and helps you to commit yourself to strengthening your conviction in it, so that you can feel healthy envy rather than unhealthy envy.

Dorothy questioned her rational belief – 'I would have much preferred it if my friend had not got the position that I coveted and deserved to get and that I had got it myself, but sadly there is no reason why this had to occur, and while it is bad that it didn't, it isn't awful' – in the following ways:

Question: Is this belief helpful or unhelpful?
Answer: It is helpful. If I believe this then I will feel healthily envious, which will (1) encourage me to understand from an objective point of view why my friend may have got the position and I didn't, and (2) motivate me to work harder and more efficiently to increase the chances of getting what I want.

Question: Is this belief true or false?
Answer: It is true. I can prove that I would have preferred to have got the position over my friend. This is my desire and it exists in me. I can also prove that there is no law of the universe that decrees that I absolutely should have got it rather than her. As I said before, if there was such a law I would have had to have got the position. I didn't, so my belief that there is no law which states that I absolutely should have got it is true.

Also, I can prove that it is bad that I didn't get the position and she did. This being the case, I have missed out on certain advantages, which is bad. I can also prove that it isn't awful that this happened. I can point to many situations that would have been worse.

Question: Is this belief logical or illogical?
Answer: It is logical. If we take my non-dogmatic preference we can see that it is made up of two components: an asserted preference component and a negated demand component. Thus: 'It would have been desirable if I had got the position rather than her (asserted preference component), but that doesn't mean that this is the way it absolutely should have been (negated demand component).' My asserted preference component that it would have been desirable if I had got the position rather than her is not rigid, and the negated demand component that this does not mean that it absolutely should have been that way is flexible. Logically, you can derive something flexible from something non-rigid, therefore my non-dogmatic preference is logical.

If we take my non-awfulizing belief, we can see that it is also made up of two components: an asserted badness component and a negated awfulizing component. Thus: 'It is bad that she got the position and I didn't (asserted badness component), but that doesn't mean that it is awful (negated awfulizing component).' My asserted badness component that it is bad that she got the position rather than me is non-extreme, and the negated awfulizing component is also non-extreme since it recognizes that it could have been worse. Therefore my non-awfulizing belief is logical, because logically you can derive something non-extreme from something non-extreme.

Using the same three questions, query your rational belief. The more convincing your responses to these questions, the more constructive their effects will be.

Step 10: Strengthen your conviction in your rational belief

After you have gained some experience at questioning both your irrational and rational beliefs, the next step is for you to strengthen your conviction in your rational belief and at the same time weaken your conviction in your irrational belief. In this section I will describe two techniques that are designed to help you to do so. These are known as the attack–response technique and the emotive-imagery technique.

The attack–response technique

The main purpose of the attack–response technique is for you to gain practice at strengthening your conviction in your rational belief by attacking it with irrational arguments, and by responding to these attacks with rational counterarguments until you have silenced the part of you that generates the irrational arguments. Here is a set of instructions for how to use the attack–response technique:

1 Write down your rational belief on a piece of paper and rate your present level of conviction in this belief next to it using a 100-point scale where 0 = no conviction and 100 = complete conviction.

2 Respond to this rational belief with an attack that is directed at this belief. This may take the form of a doubt, reservation or objection to the rational belief and should contain an irrational belief. Make this attacking statement as genuinely as you can. The more it reflects what you actually believe, the better. Write down this attack underneath the rational belief.

3 Respond to this attack as comprehensively as you can. It is particularly important that you respond to each element of the attack. Do so as persuasively as possible and write down this response underneath the first attack.

4 Continue in this vein until you have answered all your attacks and cannot think of any more.

If you find this exercise difficult, you may find it easier to make your attacks gently at first. Then, when you find that you can respond to these attacks quite easily, begin to make the attacks more pressing. Work in this way until you are making really strong attacks. When you make an attack, do so as if you really want to believe it. And when you respond, really throw yourself into your response with the intention of demolishing the attack and raising your level of conviction in your rational belief.

One important point worth stressing: the purpose of this technique is to strengthen your conviction in your rational belief. Thus, it is important that you stop only when you have answered all your attacks.

When you have answered all your attacks and cannot think of any more, write out your original rational belief and re-rate your level of conviction using the 100-point scale as before. You should find that your conviction rating has increased.

Here is how Dorothy used the attack–response technique:

Rational belief: Although I deserved to get the position that my friend got, sadly that does not mean that I had to get what I wanted.
[Conviction rating of rational belief = 40 per cent]

Attack: But it's not fair and it absolutely should not be that way. You absolutely should have got what you deserved.
Response: Well, it may not be fair, but if there was a law of the universe that decreed that I must be treated fairly then I would be treated fairly. That obviously didn't happen, and if

I continue to tell myself that it absolutely should have done it won't change anything and I'll give myself the additional unfairness of psychological disturbance.

Attack: But you sound as if it doesn't matter that you didn't get the position. Let's face it, it was terrible that you were passed over after all the work you have done.

Response: I am not saying that it doesn't matter that I didn't get what I have worked hard for. It does matter, but that isn't the same as saying that it's awful that I didn't get it. It's a pain, I admit, but awful? It's a very long way from that.

Attack: But you really wanted that position and you worked so hard for it. It didn't mean as much to your friend. She absolutely shouldn't have got. You should have.

Response: Yes, I really wanted it, and yes, I worked hard for it, but this is not the planet Dorothy. I had no divine right to get the position just because of the strength of my desire and the amount of work that I did. On the planet Earth there are other considerations, like who my employer thinks is the best person for the position. Even if the position doesn't mean as much to my friend as it does to me, that doesn't mean that I must get it rather than her. If that was the case it would have happened, and it didn't. Too bad! I don't like it, but I can definitely see that it isn't the end of the world.
[Conviction rating of original rational belief = 70 per cent]

The emotive-imagery technique

The second technique that I will describe involves the use of imagery, or the pictures that you generate in your mind. Don't be unduly concerned if you cannot get clear mental pictures; the emotive-imagery technique works whether you get clear images or not. This is how you use the emotive-imagery technique:

1 Identify a specific event about which you felt unhealthy envy.
2 Close your eyes and vividly imagine this event, focusing on

the aspect of the event that you felt most unhealthily envious about. This is known as the 'A'.

3 Deliberately rehearse the irrational belief that led you to feel unhealthy envy.

4 Allow yourself really to feel unhealthily envious while focusing on the 'A' in your mind's eye.

5 While still imagining the 'A', change your irrational belief to your rational belief and stay with this new belief until you experience healthy envy.

6 Keep with this rational belief and your feelings of healthy envy for about five minutes, all the time imagining the 'A' part of the event. If you go back to your former irrational belief, bring the rational one back.

7 Practise this technique three times a day and see what difference this makes to your level of conviction in your rational belief, which again should have increased.

Step 11: Act on your new rational belief

One of the best ways of internalizing your new rational belief so that you really believe it is to act on this belief. You need to select those behaviours that would be consistent with your rational belief and to practise them regularly. Guard against your tendency to go back to acting in ways that are consistent with your rational belief. It may help if you repeat your rational belief while you act in ways that are consistent with it. I suggest that you reread Chapter 3, where I discuss behaviours that stem from and are thus consistent with healthy envy-related rational beliefs.

Dorothy gave up all of her devised strategies to sabotage her friend and instead developed a plan to make progress in her own career. This behaviour was consistent with her developing rational belief.

Step 12: Question the thinking consequences of your unhealthy envy-based irrational belief

In Chapter 2, I discussed how unhealthy envy-related irrational beliefs affect the way that you subsequently think. At this point, it is important that you stand back and consider how realistic these thoughts are. Feeling healthily envious rather than unhealthily envious will help you to do this.

It is important that you question such thoughts rather than regard them as statements. They are inferences that stem from the irrational beliefs that underpin unhealthy envy. I recommend that you question these thoughts after, rather than before, you have challenged your irrational beliefs and you will thus be able to see that your rational beliefs are helpful, true and logical. I recommend this order because this type of thinking stems from your irrational beliefs. In other words, it occurs at 'C' in the ABC framework and stems from beliefs at 'B'.

However, you can question such thoughts before you challenge your irrational beliefs. Or you might experiment with both orders and see which one is the more helpful to you from a long-term perspective. Whichever order you select, the type of questions you can employ is the same. Here are some examples:

- Is my thinking realistic here? If not, what is a more realistic way of viewing the situation?
- How likely is it that my inference is true? If it is unlikely to be true, what inference is most likely to be true?
- Would 12 objective judges who had access to all relevant data agree that my inference is correct? If not, what would they conclude is most likely to be true?
- If I asked someone whom I could trust to give me an objective opinion about the truth or falsity of my inference, what would this person say to me and why? How would this person encourage me to view the situation instead?

- If someone told me that he or she had made this inference about the same situation and I knew all relevant data, what would I say to this person about the validity of that inference and why? How would I encourage the person to view the situation instead?

In Dorothy's case, her feelings of unhealthy envy and the irrational beliefs that underpinned them led her to think that it was grossly unfair that her friend got the position that she coveted and deserved. After she challenged her irrational belief and increased conviction in her rational belief, she recognized that while it was still somewhat unfair, it was hardly a gross unfairness. She could see that her friend had worked hard herself and also deserved promotion.

I argued above that acting in ways that are consistent with your healthy envy-related rational beliefs is a powerful way of strengthening your conviction in these rational beliefs. Additionally, if you can think realistically as you undertake such actions then you will help yourself to strengthen your conviction in these rational beliefs even further.

Step 13: Reconsider your 'A'

You will recall that in Step 5 I asked you to identify what you felt most unhealthily envious about in the episode that you chose to analyse. I also urged you to assume that it was true that your friend or family member had what you prized, but did not possess. I encouraged you to do this to identify the irrational beliefs that lay at the core of your feelings of unhealthy envy. If you had checked to see whether or not your friend or family member had what you prized but lacked, or, if they did have it, whether or not you really wanted the 'object', then you might have stopped feeling unhealthily envious (1) if you discovered the other person did not have what you thought he or she had or (2) if you discovered the other person did have it, but on reflection you didn't really want it. However, if you managed to overcome your feelings of unhealthy envy by using one of the above strategies, then you would have changed your feelings without identifying, challenging and changing the irrational beliefs that really determined your unhealthy envy. In REBT, we call this changing 'A' rather than changing 'B'. If you had bypassed your irrational beliefs at that point, you would still be vulnerable to feeling unhealthily envious about the event in question if you later thought that your inference was correct in the first place. In addition, if you had challenged your 'A' without first questioning your irrational beliefs, your challenge of 'A' would have been coloured by the ongoing existence of these irrational beliefs and would thus not be objective.

You are in a much better position, therefore, to question your 'A' that (1) your friend or family member had what you prized but lacked, and/or that (2) the 'object' that you coveted was something that had true value to you (either in terms of its usefulness to you or its ability to bring you long-term pleasure), *after* you have challenged and changed your irrational beliefs. Doing so will help you to be more objective in your questioning of 'A'. Putting this differently, feeling healthily envious will help you to stand back and take an objective view about 'A', while feeling unhealthily envious will interfere with your objectivity.

When you come to challenge your 'A', ask yourself the same questions that I outlined in Step 12 above.

Feeling healthily envious rather than unhealthily envious in the episode that she chose to analyse helped Dorothy to be objective about her inference: 'My friend got the position that I coveted and deserved to get.' She still considered that she deserved to get the position, but also recognized that her friend deserved to get it as well and that in life someone has to miss out. The work that she did on overcoming her situationally based unhealthy envy helped her to see that she is not exempt from being the one who misses out.

In this chapter, I have discussed the 13 steps that you need to take to overcome your feelings of situationally based unhealthy envy. In the next chapter, I will offer you some guidance about what you need to do in order to become less prone to unhealthy envy.

5

How to become less prone to unhealthy envy

Introduction

This is chapter is written for you if you are particularly prone to unhealthy envy and wish to become less prone to this destructive emotion. The following 21 steps are designed to help you become less prone to unhealthy envy.

Acknowledge that you are prone to unhealthy envy and that it is a problem for you

Once you have understood the nature of unhealthy envy (see Chapter 2 for a review) you have to do two things before you proceed. First, you have to decide whether you are prone to unhealthy envy – rereading pp. 31–3 will be particularly helpful here. If you are so prone, the second step is for you to decide whether this is a problem for you that you would like to change. With respect to this second point, take a sheet of paper and write down the advantages and disadvantages of experiencing unhealthy envy, both from a short-term and a long-term perspective. In doing so, review times when you have experienced unhealthy envy and remember what were the consequences of doing so. If you do this exercise thoroughly, you will in all probability conclude that the disadvantages of experiencing unhealthy envy clearly outweigh any advantages.

Once you have listed the advantages and disadvantages of your unhealthy envy, you may find it helpful to question whether or not its advantages are really beneficial, particularly from a long-term perspective. If you are unsure, ask yourself whether you would counsel somebody that you care for to experience unhealthy envy for the reason that you see as an advantage. Even if there are some benefits, recognize that you may derive these from experiencing healthy envy without incurring the costs of unhealthy envy. Thus, unhealthy envy may motivate you to get what you covet, but healthy envy will do this as well without getting you into trouble, something that may well happen if you are motivated by unhealthy envy. In this latter respect, you may find it useful to review the behavioural consequences of unhealthy envy and healthy envy in Chapters 2 and 3 respectively.

Take responsibility for being prone to unhealthy envy

You may accept that you are prone to unhealthy envy and see clearly that it is a problem for you which you would like to change, but unless you take responsibility for being prone to unhealthy envy, then you will not be effective in becoming less prone to it. Taking responsibility for your unhealthy envy means fully acknowledging that, while being deprived of what you want when friends and family members have that 'object' contributes to your feeling unhealthy envy, this deprivation does not and cannot, on its own, cause you to feel unhealthily envious. Rather, it is the irrational beliefs that you hold about this state of affairs that largely explain why you feel unhealthy envy. Taking responsibility for being prone to unhealthy envy means fully acknowledging that you hold such irrational beliefs in a variety of different situations and/or about a large number of your friends and family.

Taking such responsibility is an important step in becoming less prone to unhealthy envy. Without making this step you will continue to be prone to unhealthy envy because you will have done nothing to change the irrational beliefs that underpin your proneness.

Acknowledge that healthy envy is the constructive alternative to unhealthy envy

Once you have taken responsibility for your proneness to unhealthy envy and wish to overcome it, the next step is for you to set an appropriate goal for change. It is no good working to overcome your feelings of unhealthy envy unless you have a clear idea of what you are going to experience instead and acknowledge that this alternative emotion is acceptable to you. If either of these two conditions is absent then you will make it much harder for yourself to become less prone to unhealthy envy. Thus, if you cannot see any constructive alternative to unhealthy envy you will tend to think that you are bound to experience it. If you see that healthy envy is *an* alternative to unhealthy envy but not an acceptable one, then you will not work towards experiencing it.

Before you take this step, review Chapter 3, which is devoted to outlining the nature of healthy envy. Then, when you are clear that you have understood why healthy envy is constructive for you, take another sheet of paper and write down the advantages and disadvantages of experiencing healthy envy, again from both a short-term and a long-term perspective. In doing so, review those occasions when you experienced unhealthy envy, but this time imagine that you experienced healthy envy instead (use the material in Chapter 3 if you get stuck). Particularly, focus on the consequences of this alternative emotion.

Once you have compiled this list, you will probably conclude that experiencing healthy envy is a plausible and constructive alternative to experiencing unhealthy envy. You will probably see that what you thought were disadvantages of healthy envy are nothing of the sort; if you still think they are disadvantages, seeing the total picture will help you to realize that the existence of these disadvantages is not a stumbling block to working towards experiencing healthy envy.

Commit yourself to becoming healthily envious

After you have fully understood that healthy envy is the constructive alternative to unhealthy envy, it is important that you make a commitment to work towards experiencing this emotion when you face a situation where friends and family members have what you covet, but lack. You may find it helpful to make a written commitment to this effect and to review this every day. Also, you might consider telling someone that you are going to work towards experiencing healthy envy rather than unhealthy envy, if you consider that this verbal commitment will help you to do the work necessary to achieve your goal.

Accept yourself for being prone to unhealthy envy

One of the major obstacles to capitalizing on your commitment to become less prone to unhealthy envy at this point may be your attitude of self-depreciation for being prone to unhealthy envy. When you do this, you rate your entire 'self' on the basis of this proneness. Doing so will distract you from working to overcome your envy problem and will lead you to feel an unhealthy negative emotion such as shame. Depreciating yourself for being prone to unhealthy envy has two main effects. It does nothing to make you any less prone to this destructive emotion and gives you two emotional problems for the price of one: your original unhealthy envy, and shame for experiencing such envy.

If this applies to you, it is important that you work towards accepting yourself for being prone to unhealthy envy. You do this by seeing that your proneness does not define your 'self', but is a part of your fallibility and complexity as a human being.

Accepting yourself for being prone to unhealthy envy will enable you to focus on the factors that make you thus prone and will encourage you to do something constructive about it (like following the guidelines in this chapter) rather than resign yourself to it. Self-acceptance, therefore, promotes constructive action and discourages passivity and resignation.

Keep working on specific episodes of unhealthy envy

In the previous chapter, I outlined the steps that you need to take when working on specific episodes of unhealthy envy. In particular, I showed you how to identify what you are most unhealthily envious about and how to assess, challenge and change the irrational beliefs that underpin your situationally based unhealthy envy. I recommend that you implement this strategy as soon as you notice that you are making yourself unhealthily envious. Initially, you will need to do this on paper, but after much practice you will be able to do it in your head. You will also be more able to anticipate situations in which you are likely to make yourself unhealthily envious and deal productively with your unhealthy envy-related irrational beliefs before they take hold and lead to feelings of unhealthy envy.

Identify and make use of recurring patterns in your specific examples of unhealthy envy

Once you have worked through a number of specific examples of your unhealthy envy, you will be able to identify recurring patterns in these specific examples. Thus, you may find that your unhealthy envy is mainly object-focused. If so, make a note of the 'objects' that you feel unhealthily envious about when friends and family members have them and you don't. Or you may find that your unhealthy envy is largely person-focused, in which case make a note of which friends and/or family members you particularly envy. Also, is your unhealthy envy largely ego-based or non-ego-based?

Once you have identified recurring patterns in the specific episodes that you have worked on, you can use this information in two main ways. First, you can utilize this information when you work to prevent the occurrence of unhealthy envy in vulnerable situations, and second, this information will come in handy when you come to identify the general irrational beliefs that help to explain why you are prone to unhealthy envy.

Identify, challenge and change your general unhealthy envy-related irrational beliefs

General unhealthy envy-related irrational beliefs are irrational beliefs that are general in nature and account for your feelings of unhealthy envy across situations. Let me give you some common examples of such beliefs:

- I must have certain 'objects' that friends and family members have that I lack, and if I don't it proves that I am worthless.
- I must have certain 'objects' that friends and family members have that I lack, and I couldn't bear the deprivation if I didn't have them.
- I must have what specific friends and/or family members have that I lack, and if I don't it proves that they are more worthwhile than I am.
- I must have what specific friends and/or family members have that I lack, and if I don't then I won't be able to bear the unfairness.

You challenge your general irrational beliefs in the same way as you learned to challenge your specific irrational beliefs. Thus, you take one of your general irrational beliefs and ask yourself and answer the following questions:

- Is this belief helpful or unhelpful?
- Is this belief true or false?
- Is this belief sensible or nonsensical?

At this point, you may find it beneficial to review the material on challenging specific irrational beliefs which can be found on pp. 69–71. Continue this line of questioning until you clearly understand that your general irrational beliefs are unconstructive, false and nonsensical.

Next, develop rational alternatives to these general irrational beliefs, as follows:

- I would like to have certain 'objects' that friends and family members have that I lack, but it isn't absolutely necessary for me to have them. If I don't have them, it does not prove that I am worthless. It proves that I am a fallible human being whose worth does not depend on having what I want.
- I would like to have certain 'objects' that friends and family members have that I lack, but it isn't necessary for me to have them. If I don't have them then the deprivation is difficult to bear, but I can stand it and it will be worth bearing for my mental health.
- I would like to have what specific friends and/or family members have that I lack, but it isn't necessary for me to do so. If I don't, it does not prove that they are more worthwhile than me. It proves that we are equal in worth, but unequal in certain specific respects.
- I would like to have what specific friends and/or family members have that I lack, but it isn't necessary for me to do so. If I don't, then this unfairness will be difficult for me to tolerate, but I can do so and it will be worth it for me to do so

because it will help me either to seek fairness or to constructively adjust to it if it continues.

Once you have developed general rational beliefs, question them in the same way as you questioned your general irrational beliefs. Do this until you clearly understand that your general rational beliefs are constructive, true and logical.

Once you have done this, I suggest that you use the attack–response technique to deepen your conviction in your general rational beliefs (see pp. 73–5 for instructions concerning how to implement this technique).

Accept yourself when others have what you covet

If you are particularly prone to unhealthy ego envy, then it is important that you strive towards unconditional self-acceptance. You should do this whether your ego-based unhealthy envy is predominantly object-focused or predominantly person-focused.

Self-acceptance in object-focused healthy envy

If your ego-based unhealthy envy is predominantly object-focused, then you think that you are less worthy if friends and/or family members have 'objects' that you covet, but lack. In this type of unhealthy envy your focus is on one or more of the following: a material possession or possessions; some aspect of lifestyle (including wealth); a personality characteristic; a physical characteristic; a relationship or relationships; social attention and/or recognition; public awards or honours; and status and/or power. If you recall, I refer to the above as 'objects'.

An example of this type of ego-based unhealthy envy is Samuel, who is bald and feels envy when he sees any male friend or family member with a full head of hair. Samuel experiences unhealthy envy towards these male friends and family members for having hair which he lacks, believing that he is less worthy than they are because he doesn't have hair and they do.

The converse of this type of unhealthy envy is that you tend to think that you would be worthwhile if you got what you covet, but don't have. For example, if Samuel suddenly got a full head of hair, he would think of himself as more worthwhile than he was without hair. You may even think that you can get rid of your 'feelings' of worthlessness if you eradicate your deprivation by taking away, spoiling or rubbishing the coveted 'object' 'possessed' by a friend or family member (Samuel might go around saying how ridiculous his friend's hair looked, for example, when in reality it was the focus of his unhealthy envy).

In order to become less prone to this type of unhealthy envy it is important that you do some or all of the following:

- Show yourself that having or not having certain coveted 'objects' is not actually related to human worth unless you choose to make it a worth issue.
- Put somewhat differently, having what you covet may be worthwhile but this does not make you a worthwhile person, and while not having what you covet may be less worthwhile for you, this does not make you a less worthwhile person. Your worth as a person is constant, whereas your possession of coveted 'objects' is variable.
- As a human being you have great complexity and your worth as a person should reflect this. When you think you are more worthwhile if you have a coveted 'object' or less worthwhile if you lack this 'object', then you are not doing justice to your complexity.
- When you rate yourself on the basis of an aspect of yourself, you are making the part–whole error. This is where you use your rating of an aspect of yourself (in Samuel's case, whether or not he has hair) as a rating of your whole 'self' (in Samuel's

case, whether he is more or less worthwhile as a person). When you accept yourself, you do not make the part–whole error because you acknowledge that whether or not you possess a coveted 'object' only proves that you are the same person who either has or does not have that coveted 'object'.

- Once you base your worth on having a coveted 'object', you feel temporarily good about yourself when you obtain this 'object', but as soon as you focus on something else that you covet but don't have, you will go back to 'feeling' less worthwhile about yourself as long as you base your worth on 'object' possession. However, if you accept yourself, you are far less vulnerable in this respect.

Self-acceptance in person-focused healthy envy

If your ego-based unhealthy envy is predominantly person-focused, then you think that you are less worthy if specific friends and/or family members have what you covet, but lack. Here, your focus is more on the friend and/or family member having what you don't have than it is on the specific 'objects' themselves. Once again, you think that you can raise your worth by getting what the friend and/or family member has or by taking it away so that he or she doesn't have it, spoiling it for the person or by rubbishing that person or what he or she has. In this way, you think that you can make yourself equal to the other person with respect to worth.

In order to become less prone to this type of unhealthy envy it is important that you do some or all of the following:

- Show yourself that all humans are complex – and too complex to be given a global rating, Thus, the only sensible position to take on human worth is to see yourself as equal in worth to other people (in this case your friends and/or family members). This means that the reasons that you evaluated yourself as less worthwhile than those whom you unhealthily envy are not valid.

- Friends and/or family members whom you unhealthily envy may have 'objects' that you lack, and in fact you may never possess these 'objects'. The notion of equal worth for all humans doesn't mean that you are equal in all respects. You are as worthwhile as those whom you unhealthily envy, even though they may be better than you in a number of respects.

- If you succeed in taking away, spoiling or rubbishing what the unhealthily envied friend or family member has, this does not solve your worth problem. Although you may feel better in the short term, you have only perpetuated your worth problem and thus made it more likely that you will experience unhealthy envy of your friend or family member in the future. This is because you have reinforced the philosophy of unequal worth. If you spoil things for your friend or family member and you lose your 'feelings' of unworthiness in the process, it is only because you are saying to yourself something like, 'I am no longer less worthy than X because I have taken away from X what he or she valued and I didn't have.' In doing so, you are implying that if X still had the 'object' then you would be still be less worthwhile than X in your own mind. If you see yourself and your friend or family member as equal in worth, then you will not threatened by him or her having what you lack, but covet.

If you would like to know a lot more about developing self-acceptance, then I suggest that you consult my book on the subject, *How to Accept Yourself* (Sheldon Press, 1999).

Raise your frustration tolerance when you don't get what you want

If you are particularly prone to unhealthy non-ego envy, then it is important that you raise your frustration tolerance for not having what you want. You should do this whether your non-ego based unhealthy envy is predominantly object-focused or predominantly person-focused.

Whether your non-ego-based unhealthy envy is predominantly object-focused or predominantly person-focused, you think that you can't bear not having what friends and/or family members have in general or what specific friends and/or family members have. In this type of unhealthy envy, your focus is either on the 'object' that you covet but don't have, or on the friend or family member who has something that you don't have. An example of this type of unhealthy envy (object-focused) would be where I think that I can't bear the fact that my friend owns a laptop which I covet but cannot afford.

The converse of this type of unhealthy envy would be where you think that if you get your coveted 'object' then life will be bearable or even wonderful. Particularly if your non-ego unhealthy envy concerned the unfairness of not having what you covet when a friend and/or family member has it, you may think that you can get rid of this intolerable or unfairness by taking away, spoiling or rubbishing the coveted 'object' 'possessed' by your friend or family member. Thus, under the influence of this type of unhealthy envy, I might 'accidentally on purpose' spill coffee over my friend's laptop to get rid of the intolerable inequity of not having what I covet when my friend has it.

In order to become less prone to this type of unhealthy envy it is important that you do some or all of the following:

- Show yourself that having or not having certain coveted

'objects' is bad and difficult to tolerate but certainly not intolerable, unless you choose to view it in these terms.

- Acknowledge the grim fact that just because you want something it doesn't follow that you must get it, even though there may be many reasons it would be good for you to have it.
- Accept but do not like the fact that while it may be unfair for friends and/or family members to have what you covet but don't have, you are not exempt from experiencing such unfairness. If you accept this, then you will also see that in other areas you benefit from unfairness, meaning that you have what they don't have but covet. Acknowledge that your life is made up of fairness (where you get what you deserve); two types of unfairness: (1) where you don't get what you deserve and (2) where you get what you don't deserve; and serendipity (where you get or don't get things independently of whether you deserve them or not).

If you would like to know a lot more about developing high frustration tolerance, then I suggest that you consult a book on the subject that I wrote with Jack Gordon, *Beating the Comfort Trap* (Sheldon Press, 1993).

Develop a healthy attitude towards 'objects'

Throughout this book, I have spoken about 'objects'. When I have done so I have placed inverted commas around the word because I wish to denote that it stands for a variety of different things that human beings envy (whether unhealthily or healthily). These different things include: material possessions; some aspects of lifestyle (including wealth); personality characteristics; physical characteristics; relationships; social attention and/or recognition; public awards or honours; and status and/or power.

As part of a package of measures to help you become less

prone to unhealthy envy, I suggest that you rethink your view of the place of such 'objects' in your life and think about developing a healthy attitude to having such 'objects'. In doing so, I suggest that you consider the following:

- Are the 'objects' that you covet truly necessary in your life, or would they enhance your life in some way but not be necessary to it? Remember that if something is necessary you literally cannot do without it, even if you hold a healthy set of beliefs about not having it.
- How important are such 'objects' in your life compared to friends, family, children? Bizarre as it may sound for me to even suggest it, would you sacrifice the health of a loved one if you could get coveted 'objects'? If not, why not? Write down as many reasons as possible why you would refuse these 'objects' to safeguard the health of your loved one (assuming that you would, of course). What does this say about your true attitude to the place of coveted 'objects' in your life?
- If you were to give your children (present or future) advice about the role of 'objects' in their lives, what would that advice be? Would you say to a daughter, for example: 'Don't forget, being attractive is the only thing that matters in life. If you lose your looks, your life is over'? If not, why not? And if you wouldn't say that to a child, why persist in saying such a thing to yourself?

If you redefine the place of 'objects' in your life and give them due importance but not undue unimportance, then you will help yourself become less prone to unhealthy envy.

At a time when you are not feeling unhealthy envy, identify the 'objects' that you envy and ask yourself why you really want them

If you are particularly prone to unhealthy envy, you will probably have noticed one interesting phenomenon. When you feel unhealthily envious about not having what you covet while a friend or family member does have this 'object', you often become preoccupied with that 'object' and think how great it is and how much better your life would be if you had it. Then, if you manage to get the coveted 'object', reality kicks in: you notice that the 'object' isn't as great as you thought it would be and that your life doesn't change appreciably for the better. You then put aside the 'object', since it hasn't lived up to its promise.

When you are particularly prone to unhealthy envy your irrational beliefs are core in nature, which means that, among other things, you tend to experience it across a range of situations. Given this, you will soon find another 'object' that someone else has which you covet but lack. You then bring your unhealthy envy-related irrational beliefs to this new situation and once again you idealize the new coveted 'object', become preoccupied with it and think that your life would change for the better if you possessed it. When you do possess it, reality kicks in again and you are disappointed to find that the new 'object' doesn't fulfil your fantasy. So you turn the wheel again, cast this 'object' aside and focus on yet another new coveted 'object' which this time will be the one to change your life.

In breaking this vicious circle, you need to do a number of things which I have either already discussed in this chapter or soon will. Thus, you need to identify, challenge and change your core unhealthy envy-related irrational beliefs, and every time you become preoccupied with an 'object' trace this thinking back to the irrational beliefs that have spawned your preoccupation and challenge them. You also need to stop taking action that is designed to obtain the 'object' of your unhealthy envy unless you have clear evidence that you will use and value the 'object' and will not cast it aside. In order to do this you need to consider each 'object' that you envy and, when you are not feeling unhealthily envious, you need to list the reasons it is healthy for you to pursue it. If you cannot see yourself getting ongoing use and/or pleasure from it, then it is something not worth pursuing.

Make the following a guiding principle: pursue an 'object' only when you are convinced that you will get ongoing use and/or pleasure from it. If you think that it will change your life substantially, you are operating under an unhealthy illusion and it is best not to pursue the 'object' in question, but to identify, challenge and change the unhealthy envy-related irrational belief that, in all probability, has produced this illusion.

Appreciate that general unhealthy envy-related irrational beliefs lead you to focus on what you don't have and that general healthy envy-related rational beliefs lead to a balanced view of what you have and don't have in life

As I discussed in Chapter 2 and reiterated earlier in this chapter, one of the effects of holding unhealthy envy-related irrational beliefs is on your subsequent thinking. When you hold *general* unhealthy envy-related irrational beliefs, these general irrational beliefs affect your thinking across the board rather than just in specific situations. One of the general thinking effects of holding general unhealthy envy-related irrational beliefs is that they lead you to focus on what you don't have in life. This means that, as you go about your daily business, you are likely to be particularly attentive to 'objects' that you covet but don't possess, and when you focus on these particular 'objects' you evaluate them using a specific form of your general unhealthy envy-related irrational belief.

On the other hand, when you change your general unhealthy envy-related irrational beliefs to general healthy envy-related rational beliefs, the effect that this has is to make you more balanced in your thinking. Instead of being particularly sensitive to situations in which other people have what you don't have but covet (whether you truly want these 'objects' or not), you are aware of both what you lack in life and what you have. In addition, when you hold healthy envy-related rational beliefs you are likely to be envious of 'objects' that you are likely to use and/or *enjoy* for a long time and that you will not cast aside after a brief period of time.

So, another way of helping yourself to be less prone to unhealthy envy is this: after you have challenged your unhealthy envy-related irrational beliefs and are beginning to look at relevant events through the lens of your healthy envy-related rational beliefs, make a deliberate effort to remind yourself of what you do have in your life as well as what you don't have. If you can appreciate what you have as well, then this will also help to counter your tendency to focus on what you don't have and to covet such 'objects'.

Practise healthy action and thinking tendencies and limit unhealthy tendencies

Identify the action and thinking tendencies based on your unhealthy envy-related irrational beliefs and develop a list of alternative healthy action and thinking tendencies based on your general healthy envy-related rational beliefs. Resolve to practise the latter and limit the former.

In Chapter 2, I emphasized the fact that when you hold

unhealthy envy-related irrational beliefs, these beliefs have an effect on the way that you subsequently tend to think and act. If you turn these tendencies into actualities then you strengthen your conviction in these irrational beliefs and make yourself more prone to experience unhealthy envy.

In Chapter 3, on the other hand, I stressed that when you hold healthy envy-related irrational beliefs, then these beliefs have a different and more constructive effect on the way that you subsequently tend to think and act. If you turn these tendencies into actualities then you strengthen your conviction in these rational beliefs and make yourself less prone to experience unhealthy envy.

Following on from the above, I suggest that you act as follows:

- Develop a list of the ways in which you tend to think and act once you feel unhealthily envious.
- Become aware of times when you experience the tendency to think and act in the above ways and resist doing so. Instead, use these tendencies to go back to challenge the unhealthy envy-related irrational beliefs that spawned them.
- Develop a list of the ways in which you would tend to think and act if you held healthy envy-related irrational beliefs. These should be constructive alternatives to the thinking and action tendencies that you listed at the beginning of this exercise.
- Once you have challenged your unhealthy envy-related irrational beliefs and have begun to hold the rational alternatives to these beliefs, encourage yourself to think and act in ways that are consistent with the thinking and action tendencies.

Thus, a powerful way of making yourself less prone to unhealthy envy is to hold rational beliefs at the same time as you think and act in ways that reinforce such beliefs. If you hold healthy envy-related rational beliefs but think and act in ways that are consistent with the unhealthy envy-related irrational beliefs, you will tend to go back to these latter beliefs and spoil the work that you are trying to do to make yourself less prone to unhealthy envy. Thus, guard against doing this.

Develop and rehearse a view of the world founded on healthy envy-related rational beliefs

In my book *How to Make Yourself Miserable* (Sheldon Press, 2001), I show that when you are prone to unhealthy envy you operate on a view of the world that is founded on the irrational beliefs that underpin this emotion. In Chapter 2, I discussed the elements of this world view in unhealthy envy and how they influence the inferences that you make. Consequently, in order to become less prone to unhealthy envy, it is important that you develop a world view founded on healthy envy-related rational beliefs. The following are the major components of the healthy envy-based world view with, in brackets, the inferences that you will tend to make when you operate on this world view:

- The grass is sometimes greener in the lives of friends and family members, but not always. (Sometimes what I have is less attractive than what friends and/or family members have, but at other times what I have is more attractive.)
- Satisfaction can be achieved even if I don't get what I want. (If I get what I covet it may satisfy me if it is what I really want.)
- It's unfair if friends and family members have what I don't have only if I truly deserve to have it, and it is unfair if I have what others don't have only if they truly deserve to have it. Life is comprised of fairness and unfairness. (If I don't have something that I covet but lack, this inequality is unfair only if I deserve to have it.)
- People's worth is defined by their aliveness, humanity and uniqueness, not by what they have in life. (Some people may

like me more if I have a lot in my life than if I have a little, but others will like me for who I am rather than what I have.)

- Happiness occurs when I am striving to reach personally meaningful goals rather than when I get what I want. (In some situations it is better to have what I don't have than to be content with what I do have, but in other situations I can be happy if I don't have what I covet, if I am engaged in the pursuit of personally meaningful goals.)

Accept that, in all probability, friends and family members will, in some area, always have what you don't have and covet, and acknowledge that you don't have to get rid of this inequality

A major component of unhealthy envy is a sense of inequality (that a friend and/or family member has what you don't have, but covet) and a belief that you must get rid of this inequality, either by getting what the friend has, for example, or by taking it away from the person, spoiling it for him or her or rubbishing the coveted 'object' or the friend who has it.

Given this, you can become less prone to unhealthy envy in two ways. First, accept the grim reality that in all probability others will, in some area of life, have what you don't have but covet. Second, develop and hold the general rational belief that while you may want this inequality not to exist, you don't have to have your desire met. Consequently, you don't have to take steps to get rid of this inequality, although at times, when you really want the coveted 'object' and it is feasible for you to get it, then it is sensible for you to take such steps.

This dual approach of accepting grim reality and flexibly pursuing what you covet but don't have will go a long way to helping you to become less prone to unhealthy envy if you rehearse it and act on it.

Develop a healthy perspective on making comparisons

Another major component of unhealthy envy is the making of unhealthy comparisons. This is particularly the case in unhealthy ego envy. When you make an unhealthy comparison in unhealthy ego envy you compare your situation with that of another person and you conclude two things:

1 This person has what I don't have and covet.
2 This person is worthier than me (or superior to me) for having the coveted 'object'.

In order to become less prone to unhealthy envy, continue to make the first comparison, but not the second. Thus, compare your situation with that of the other and conclude:

1 This person has what I don't have and covet.
2 This person is neither worthier than me nor superior to me for having what I covet, but lack. We are both equal as people, but unequal in this respect.

Put a little differently, becoming less prone to unhealthy ego envy involves you comparing your situation with that of another person when that person has what you covet, but lack, but without differentially comparing your 'self' with the 'self' of the other person.

Work on overcoming your resentment

When you are prone to unhealthy envy you are also likely to feel resentment. It follows that if you want to become less prone to unhealthy envy, it would be useful for you to overcome your feelings of resentment. Resentment is a form of unhealthy anger that you feel towards a friend and/or family member whom you consider a rival when that person has what you covet but lack, and when you believe that he or she absolutely should not have the coveted 'object' when you do not have it.

In order to overcome your feelings of resentment you need to challenge and change the above irrational belief and accept that, while you would rather your friend or family member did not have what you covet but lack, there is no law of the universe that decrees that he or she must not benefit in this way. If you do develop, practise and act on this rational belief you will overcome your feelings of resentment and become less prone to unhealthy envy as a result.

Guard against indulging in *schadenfreude*

Schadenfreude is pleasure that you experience at the hardship or suffering of others. You are particularly likely to experience *schadenfreude* if you are especially prone to person-focused unhealthy ego envy. Thus, for example, when you feel unhealthy envy towards someone to whom you 'feel' inferior, you will feel pleasure if that person experiences some misfortune. Since *schadenfreude* is a pleasurable feeling it would be easy for you to indulge in this emotion. When you do this, you maintain the irrational beliefs that underpin your unhealthy envy and thus you sustain your proneness to this disturbed emotion.

If you want to become less prone to unhealthy envy, you need to curtail your feelings of *schadenfreude* and instead use these feelings to identify, challenge and change the irrational beliefs that underpin it.

Learn about the familiarity principle and strive to go against it

The familiarity principle describes a tendency for humans to think, feel and act in ways that are familiar to them, and to seek out situations that are familiar to them as well. Thus, if you are prone to unhealthy envy you will find the feelings, thoughts and behaviours that are involved in your unhealthy envy familiar and very easy to experience, even though they are detrimental to your well-being. Thus, in order for you to become less prone to unhealthy envy you will need to tolerate the discomfort of holding healthy envy-related rational beliefs and acting and thinking in ways that are consistent with them.

Please accept the discomfort that is almost always associated with personal change, and if you find yourself setting up situations that make it likely that you will experience your old familiar feelings of unhealthy envy, realize that you are operating according to the familiarity principle. Understanding and learning from what you are doing and renewing your resolve to tolerate the unfamiliarity of personal change will help you to transcend the familiarity principle until you become used to experiencing healthy envy. In doing so, you will become less prone to unhealthy envy.

Identify what really matters in your life and actively involve yourself in these things

The final tip that I want to give you to help you to become less prone to healthy envy involves you taking a broader look at your life and identifying what really matters to you. Then, I suggest that you actively involve yourself in what you have identified. If you do this after you have challenged and changed your unhealthy envy-related irrational beliefs to their rational counterparts, then you will only pursue 'objects' that you truly covet and that will provide you with lasting use and pleasure.

If you regularly implement the 21 steps found in this chapter, you should go a long way to experiencing far less unhealthy envy than hitherto. In the final chapter we revisit the people we met in Chapter 2 and see how they overcame their problems with unhealthy envy.

6

From unhealthy envy to healthy envy: the case studies revisited

Introduction

In this final chapter, I will return to the cases of the five people I discussed in Chapter 2 whose lives were affected for the worse by unhealthy envy. In doing so, I will show how they used the principles in this book to help themselves overcome their problems of unhealthy envy. While reading each of the cases described in this chapter you may find it useful to reread the corresponding case in Chapter 2. In this way you can get more of a 'before and after' sense of the benefits of an REBT approach to unhealthy envy.

Leonard: a case of unhealthy object-focused ego envy

If you recall from Chapter 2, Leonard is a 25-year-old single man who works as a messenger for a large city firm of solicitors. He considers himself to be a man's man and likes going out with the lads and following Burnley FC, his favourite football team. Leonard has a 'macho' philosophy, where he values having a laugh with the lads, 'pulling birds', physical strength and emotional self-control. Unfortunately for Leonard, he has not been blessed with a physique to match his macho aspirations. Indeed, he is physically slight with poorly defined muscles. His friends tease him by calling him 'Skinny', which he hates, but he masks his feelings by laughing and joking in response to these teasing remarks.

Leonard experienced unhealthy object-focused ego envy about his male friends' muscular physique. His irrational belief that underpinned his envy was as follows: 'I must be muscular like my male friends and because I am not I am a weed.'

In using the principles of this book, Leonard challenged the two components of this irrational belief and developed the following rational belief: 'I would like to be muscular like my male friends, but I don't have to be this way. I am not a weed if I don't have the build that I would like to have. Rather, I am a complex fallible human being with many different and important aspects. One aspect of my complexity cannot define me as a unique person.'

As he strengthened this rational belief, Leonard became less aware of his male friends' muscular frames in comparison to his own non-muscular frame and focused more on other aspects of the men that he came into contact with. He also became more accepting of the unfairness of him not having a muscular build when his male friends had, and began to see that his life is made up of fairness and unfairness and that this is the case for all humans. In doing so, he stopped cursing his parents for being so puny themselves and accepted that, while being muscular was important to him, it wasn't the be-all and end-all that he previously thought it was. He stopped thinking that everyone considered him to be a wimp, someone to kick around if he gave them the chance, and saw that different male friends had different opinions about him based on things other than his build. These became the thinking consequences of his new healthy envy-related ego rational belief.

With respect to his behaviour, as he developed his rational belief he stopped buying body-building magazines and stopped sending away for body-building supplements. He saw both activities as helping to maintain his previously held irrational belief and thereby something to be resisted, although he did at times feel the urge to resume these activities. He used this urge to go back to identifying and challenging his underlying unhealthy envy-related ego irrational belief. He still went to the gym, but less frequently than before, and exercised within sensible limits. This cut down on the amount of money he had to spend on physiotherapy bills.

As a result of these changes, Leonard began to see that there was more to life than going out with the lads and following Burnley FC, although he still did both. He became less macho in outlook, and began to treat women with greater respect and to give more thought to what he wanted to do with his life.

Hilary: a case of unhealthy object-focused non-ego envy
If you recall, Hilary is a 32-year-old married woman who is a solicitor. She has a good job, many friends and a husband who is devoted to her. They have been married for three years and plan to have children when

Hilary is 35. Hilary has had a comfortable upbringing and has wanted for very little in her life.

Despite all of this, Hilary experienced unhealthy object-focused non-ego envy about her friends' possessions. Her irrational belief that underpinned her envy was as follows: 'I must have the possessions that my friends have and that I don't have. If I don't, then I can't bear the deprivation.'

In using the principles of this book, Hilary challenged the two components of this irrational belief and developed the following rational belief: 'I would like to have the possessions that my friends have, but it is certainly not necessary that I have them. If I don't have them, I can bear the deprivation even though it is a struggle for me to do so. It is definitely worth the effort for me to do so.'

Hilary's new rational belief led her to be less aware that her friends had possessions that she did not have, and she dwelled far less on the deprivation that she 'felt', a 'feeling' that was far less than when she held her irrational belief. Consequently, she was able to acknowledge that her life was going reasonably well. She had very few thoughts of taking the possessions away from her friends or of how she could spoil their enjoyment of them. These were the thinking consequences of her new healthy envy-related non-ego rational belief.

Behaviourally, Hilary only went out to buy the possessions that she really wanted and from which she could either get ongoing use or derive ongoing pleasure. She was thus able to pay off the debts that she had accrued when operating on her irrational belief. She also gave up prostitution (to pay for what she craved) and stealing, practices that she had involved herself in when she believed that she had to get what she coveted.

Jennifer: a case of unhealthy person-focused ego envy

If you recall, Jennifer is a 23-year-old single woman who works in an office as an admin assistant. She has a small number of good friends and a larger number of acquaintances. Jennifer has a large number of brothers and sisters and was brought up by loving parents in a working-class area.

Jennifer's unhealthy envy was ego-based person-focused, in that she harboured envious feelings towards Barbara and Betty, two of her first cousins. She envied them many things, including their boyfriends, their relationship with one another, their looks and their clothes. In comparing herself to Barbara and Betty, Jennifer invariably felt badly about herself, something she covered up with her unhealthy envy-related thinking and behaviour. The irrational belief that underpinned Jennifer's unhealthy envy was as follows: 'I must have what Barbara and Betty have. If I don't then this proves that I am inferior to them.'

In using the principles of this book, Jennifer challenged the two components of this irrational belief and developed the following rational belief: 'I would like to have what Barbara and Betty have, but I do not have to have what they have. If I lack what they have this certainly does not mean that I am inferior to them. It means that we are all equal in worth, but unequal in what we have in life.'

As she gained conviction in this rational belief, Jennifer became far less focused on Barbara and Betty and less aware of what her cousins had that she lacked. When she became aware that Barbara and Betty had 'objects' that she did not have but truly coveted, Jennifer felt healthily envious. She acknowledged that she wanted the 'objects' and thought of ways that she could get them, but she did not wish to spoil things for Barbara and Betty or take the prized 'objects' away from them. She also compared herself with her two cousins far less and did not 'feel' inferior to them. She was thus far less motivated to 'rubbish' Barbara and Betty to herself and to others, strategies she had employed when holding her irrational beliefs as a way of coping with the pain of unhealthy envy. Instead of putting their boyfriends down in her mind as being flash and chauvinistic, she admitted that she found their boyfriends attractive and that she wished she could go out with such people.

Behaviourally, Jennifer no longer spoke about Barbara and Betty in derogatory ways to other people and refrained from making up stories about them which put them in a negative light with her family or friends. She began to talk to Barbara and Betty and was able to look at them. She started to go family events attended by Barbara and Betty and was able to enjoy herself there instead of spending the evening making bitchy remarks about them to others present.

While she never became friends with Barbara and Betty, Jennifer was on speaking terms with them and she thought about them far less than before, when she held her unhealthy envy-related irrational belief.

Tom: a case of unhealthy person-focused non-ego envy

If you recall, Tom is a 43-year-old man who works as an insurance salesman. From schooldays, Tom has had a competitive relationship with Jim, a childhood friend he grew up with and still sees regularly. Tom's parents were quite poor even though they lived in a prosperous community. This was due to the fact that Tom's mother inherited the family house from her mother. Given this, Tom was aware early on in his life that his contemporaries always had more than he did. He was not unduly bothered about this, but when it came to Jim it was a different matter. According to Tom, Jim was always bragging to Tom about what he had and made fun of Tom's poor background. Tom thought that this was unfair and was determined to prove that anything Jim could have, he could have.

Tom's unhealthy envy was non-ego-based and person-focused in that he harboured envious feelings towards a given friend, Jim. However, he did not feel that he was inferior if he did not have what Jim had. Rather, he focused on the deprivation he experienced, which he believed he could not bear. The irrational belief that underpinned Tom's unhealthy envy was as follows: 'I must have what Jim has. I can't bear being deprived in this way.'

In using the principles of this book, Tom challenged the two components of this irrational belief and developed the following rational belief: 'I would like to have what Jim has, but it really isn't essential to me that I have it. If I don't have it I can truly bear the deprivation even though I will never like it, and it is worth it to me to bear it.'

Tom's rational belief allowed him to become less aware that Jim had possessions that he did not have, and when he was aware of this he spent far less time thinking about how he could get what Jim had that he lacked. He stopped thinking that it was grossly unfair that Jim had the wherewithal to have so many possessions without having to work hard for them, while he, Tom, worked his fingers to the bone and yet had little money for the luxuries in life. He began to accept that this was part of life and that there was no reason why it had to be different just because he wanted it to be different.

Behaviourally, Tom's healthy envy-related irrational belief led him to stop buying what Jim bragged about. Indeed, he acknowledged that most of the things that Jim bragged about were not what he truly wanted anyway. When he did focus on something that Jim had that he did not have but in reality truly wanted, Tom did not go into debt to get it. He asserted to himself that he didn't have to get it immediately. Rather, he would save up for it, even if it took a long time to get into his possession. In doing so, he began to learn the value of working to get something rather than getting it immediately and hang the consequences. Consequently, in doing so he began to pay off the loan shark he had unwisely borrowed from to fund procuring what he thought he needed.

Tom stopped moaning about Jim and the unfairness of the system that allowed Jim to get what he wanted without having to work for it. Consequently, he renewed his friendships and was reconciled with his family. In doing so, he realized that family and friends are far more important than the latest example of Jim's profligacy and the unfairness that surrounded it.

Samantha: a case of mixed unhealthy envy

So far I have discussed cases where the person's original unhealthy envy was fairly pure. In other words, the individual's unhealthy envy was either person-focused or object-focused and either ego or non-ego in nature. Originally, I chose to present these 'pure types' in Chapter 2 to help you understand the processes involved in unhealthy envy in a clear manner. However, in reality much unhealthy envy is mixed in nature rather than pure. This is shown in the case of Samantha that I originally discussed in Chapter 2.

If you recall, Samantha is a 45-year-old unmarried woman who works as a hardware consultant in IT. She lives alone and has few friends. She is very bright, but is quite lazy and has never fulfilled her intellectual potential. She has experienced much unhealthy envy in her life. In terms of person-focused envy she envies her two sisters who are more attractive, more successful and more popular than she is and who are both happily married with loving husbands and well-adjusted children.

Samantha's unhealthy person-focused envy was both ego and non-ego in nature. From an ego perspective, she held the following irrational belief which comprised a demand and a self-depreciation belief: 'I must have what my sisters have and if I don't then it proves that I am inferior to them as a person.'

In using the principles of this book, Samantha challenged the two components of this irrational belief and developed the following rational belief: 'I would like to have what my sisters have, but it isn't imperative for me to have it. If I don't, I'm not inferior to them as a person. We are equal in worth even though unequal in the sense that they have what I don't have in this respect.'

As her conviction in this rational belief increased, Samantha developed a more balanced view of her strengths and weaknesses. As a result, she cut down drastically on the number of telephone calls she made to her friends telling them how worthless she felt.

She also cut down on using food and drink to cope with her feelings of unhealthy envy, as she began to experience healthy envy. As a result, she lost weight and began to get her energy back so that she began to achieve more.

From a non-ego perspective, Samantha's person-focused unhealthy envy was based on the following irrational belief which comprises a demand and an awfulizing belief: 'It's unfair that my sisters have what I don't have and want and it absolutely should not be this way. It's truly awful that this unfairness exists.'

Samantha challenged the two components of this irrational belief and developed the following rational belief: 'It may be unfair that my sisters have what I don't have, but there is no reason on this earth why it must not be that way. It is that way, and while this is unfortunate it certainly isn't awful.'

As she developed this rational belief, Samantha focused less on the unfairness she has experienced in life that involved her sisters, and indeed she began to see the role that she played in her own under-achievement. This led to a different focus in counselling where she identified, challenged and changed the irrational beliefs that hindered her from fulfilling her potential in life. All this helped her to move away from crippling self-pity.

In addition to her person-focused unhealthy envy, Samantha also experienced object-focused unhealthy envy. In particular, she harboured unhealthily envious feelings towards her friends who are successful in their careers. In this respect, her ego-based object-focused unhealthy envy stemmed from the following irrational belief which comprises a demand and a self-depreciation belief: 'I must be as successful in my career as my friends are in theirs, and if I'm not then it proves that I am inadequate.'

Once again, using the principles in this book Samantha challenged this irrational belief and developed the following rational belief: 'I would like to be as successful in my career as my friends are in theirs, but unfortunately I don't have to be. If I'm not, it does not prove that I am inadequate as a person. It proves that I am a fallible human being who for whatever reason is not successful in my career.'

In the wake of this rational belief, Samantha stopped thinking that she did not have what it takes to be successful in her own career and started to look at why she wasn't, as I mentioned above. As she did so, she decided to take a risk and go back to the manager who had offered to sponsor her to go on training seminars and ask if he would give her another chance. He did and she began to revive her career, slowly but surely.

Samantha's object-focused unhealthy envy was also non-ego in nature. Here, she focused on the benefits her friends derived from being successful in their careers that she lacked by not being successful in hers.

The irrational belief that underpinned this type of unhealthy envy was comprised of a demand and a low frustration tolerance belief, as follows: 'I must have the benefits that my friends, who are successful in their careers, have, and it is unbearable that I don't.'

She challenged and changed this irrational belief to the following rational belief: 'I would prefer to have the benefits that my friends, who are successful in their careers, have, but I don't absolutely need these benefits. It is difficult to put up with not having these benefits, but I can certainly do so and it is worth doing so because it leads me to focus more on what I can do to get these benefits rather than being passive, silently feeling unhealthily envious and resentful.'

Thinking rationally in this respect, Samantha stopped daydreaming about these benefits and began to knuckle down to the hard work needed to be successful and thus to derive the benefits. She did so without self-pity and, as I mentioned above, she began to revive her stagnant career. As she did so, she began to gain benefits like those that others received for their hard work.

You have now reached the end of the book. I hope you have found it valuable, and if you would like to share your experiences of using it please write to me c/o Sheldon Press. Thank you.

Index